Natural Remedies with Essential Oils

A Hands-On Guide to DIY Beauty, Home Solutions, and Health Remedies

Natural Apothecary

Natural

Remedies

with Essential

Oils

A Hands-On Guide to DIY Beauty, Home Solutions, and Health Remedies

Natural Apothecary

The following Book is reproduced below with the goal of providing information that is as accurate and reliable as possible. Regardless, purchasing this Book can be seen as consent to the fact that both the publisher and the author of this book are in no way experts on the topics discussed within and that any recommendations or suggestions that are made herein are for entertainment purposes only. Professionals should be consulted as needed prior to undertaking any of the action endorsed herein.

This declaration is deemed fair and valid by both the American Bar Association and the Committee of Publishers Association and is legally binding throughout the United States.

Furthermore, the transmission, duplication, or reproduction of any of the following work including specific information will be considered an illegal act irrespective of if it is done electronically or in print. This extends to creating a secondary or tertiary copy of the work or a recorded copy and is only allowed with the express written consent from the Publisher. All additional right reserved.

The information in the following pages is broadly considered a truthful and accurate account of facts and as such, any inattention, use, or misuse of the information in question by the

Table of Content

Introduction

The ancient knowledge of healing and promoting health with fragrant natural ingredients called essential oils goes under the modern name of aromatherapy. These ingredients are found in herbs, plants, flowers, fruits and the bark, roots or resin of some trees.

Essential oils give a plant its fragrance, but they also contain dozens of complex chemicals that seem to do everything from beautify the skin or speed healing to induce sleep or suppress headaches.

Even if you believe you have never used these oils before, they have an impact on everyone on a daily basis.Every time you peel an orange, the essential oil releases a bittersweet, acidic citrus aroma into the air as it evaporates due to its extreme volatility. The essential oil streams out of the small pockets in the peel. And whether you know it or not, orange oil has a calming yet energizing impact.

Aromatherapy is the process of bringing flowers to a hospitalized patient to make them feel better.For instance, the compounds in lavender, jasmine, rose, and geranium essential oils help to rapidly lift one's spirits by relaxing the neurological system.

The health benefits of pure essential oils, on the other hand, are more concentrated and impact the body and mind more than those found in smelling a bouquet of flowers.Thus, mastering the usage of these essential oils will enable you to lead a healthier, happier, and more in-charge life in every aspect.

What Is An Essential Oil?

Exactly what essential oils are can be difficult to define because they are so complex and magical. They are the plant's life energy, according to romantics and enthusiasts, much like the human spirit.

According to scientists, they are a mixture of hundreds of different molecules, many of which are too small or complicated to be classified under a microscope, including ketones, terpenes, esters, alcohols, and aldehydes. Fortunately, understanding what they do is far simpler than understanding who they are.

Due to their tiny size and high volatility, essential oils can pass through the epidermis and into the bloodstream and organs before being eliminated completely. Hours after being rubbed into the skin, researchers have discovered that the same oils repeatedly accumulate in the same bodily areas.

Few objects can really pierce human skin, which is what makes them special and so healing. There is no denying essential oils' ability to cure. Scientists studying plants are discovering more and more essential components in nature instead of in test tubes these days.

For example, the pain reliever aspirin comes from the willow, the Australian tea tree contains a dozen more powerful germ killers than any other antibacterial, and good old carrots are full of beta-carotene, which has now proven to be an important weapon in battle against cancer.

Scientists are discovering new benefits in every organic chemical found in nature as they continue to research plants and their characteristics. It seems like everything has a purpose. But what really interests me is that the most recent study validates the accuracy and efficacy of the herbal traditions that healers have been using for ages.

A Little History

Humanity has had to conduct experiments with plants to determine which ones were edible and which were lethal ever since the beginning of life on Earth. Some were set aside for magic or medicine along the road, and it is from them that the numerous folk treatments originated.

Essential oils were widely used in daily life by the time the majority of ancient civilizations were flourishing. Using myrrh and cedarwood oils for embalming, the Egyptians achieved perfection 6500 years afterward, as evidenced by their flawlessly preserved mummies from 4500 BC. The reason most mummies look so young for their age is because myrrh has potent antiseptic and antibacterial properties, while cedarwood includes a natural fixative, according to recent research.

The process of distilling plants to extract their essential oils was initially used by the Egyptians. They used them for embalming, as well as for medicinal purposes, religious ceremonies, and as potions and perfumes for beautifying the skin and face. Oils were offered to the gods because they were so valuable. On papyrus scrolls, the high priests documented the therapeutic applications, recognized qualities, and coded formulae for the oils. Their expertise is so precise that it serves as the foundation for contemporary aromatherapy.

The Romans, on the other hand, took daily, leisurely, fragrant baths and massages and employed essential oils for both therapeutic and pleasurable purposes. Legend has it that Emperor Nero loved orgies, feasts, and perfumes. Rose oil was his favorite oil since it helped with stomach, headaches, and mood swings, which allowed him to continue having parties. Another favorite of the Romans was chamomile, which was used to cure wounds and treat skin conditions. It is now recognized that chamomile has a natural anti-inflammatory substance called azulene, which explains why chamomile has such a rejuvenating impact on skin.

Arabia, Greece, India, and China were all major users of aromatics. However, the practice of perfumery and herbalism did not make its way to Europe until the 12th century. It was so well-established by the time of the Great Plague in 1665 that Londoners carried posies of the same plants as their only defense against infectious sickness and burned bundles of lavender, cedar, and cypress in the streets. And since all of these plants contain potent antibacterial properties, it certainly saved thousands of lives.

Up until the turn of the century, all medications and treatments were made from plants. Herbalists and apothecaries prescribed infusions, ointments, and powders for conditions ranging from impotence to hair loss. However, "modern" medicine quickly took over, as pharmaceutical chemists produced small, miraculous tablets that rendered many natural cures outdated and archaic. By the 1960s, research into herbal remedies had fallen to secondary importance as the world's attention was directed toward advancements in surgery, hospitals, and medicine.

The term "Aromathérapie," albeit derived from more than 6000 years of knowledge, was first used almost a century ago by a French chemist by the name of Gattefossé. His family ran a perfume company. Gattefossé once severely burned his hand while working in the laboratory and submerged it in a vat of lavender essential oil. Upon the burn's speedy healing without blistering, Gattefossé developed a lifetime fascination with researching the medicinal qualities of plant oils.

Modern aromatherapy was thus created. Numerous enthusiasts have now carried out additional research, including Dr. Jean Valnet.

During World War II, Valnet treated injured soldiers with a lot of oils. But Marguerite Maury, a French biochemist, is credited with creating the technique that we now refer to as aromatherapy—which involves diluting and massaging essential oils.

The 1980s marked the advent of contemporary aromatherapy's maturity. Recently, biochemists have identified dozens of components in essential oils that are responsible for their remarkable qualities. And now that the traditional cures have been supported by empirical evidence, aromatherapy is more widely acknowledged and well-liked than ever.

Useful Details

Plant components are the source of essential oils. They appear to gather in the petals of some, and in the roots, rinds, stalks, seeds, sap, nuts, leaves, or bark of others. Only once the tree is 40 years old does sandalwood oil begin to accumulate in the heart wood of the tree. Jasmine flowers should be hand-picked before dawn to yield the best oil, as the concentrated jasmine content occurs in the petals during the night when the blooms are just one day old.

Of all the oils, rose is the rarest and priciest. One kilogram (two pounds) of essential oil is produced from two tons of fresh petals in full bloom.

Conversely, a simple orange tree yields three oils. orange oil from the fruit rind, petitgrain from the leaves, and neroli from the blossoms—each with unique qualities.

Like a good wine's vintage, the quality of an essential oil can change from year to year. Along with climate and harvest timing, altitude and soil conditions can have an impact on quality. Selecting the raw material should only be the first step; otherwise, the essential oils may not be of the highest quality if they are extracted improperly or left on for too long.

Purchasing pure essential oils from a reliable supplier is crucial since diluted or lower-quality oils may lose their effectiveness. Thankfully, due to the growing popularity of essential oils, high-quality oils can now be purchased from specialty beauty stores, mail order businesses, and health food stores around the Western world.

How Are Essential Oils Extracted?

The fact that essential oils aren't at all greasy is the biggest surprise. Most are light liquids, meaning they quickly evaporate in air but do not dissolve in water.

They are available in a variety of hues: geranium is colorless, sage is pale lime, violet is forest green, chamomile is crystal blue, and patchouli oil is plum.

Somewhere on the living plant, small sacs contain the liquid. It can be quite difficult to extract it before it escapes into the atmosphere. Steam-distilling the raw ingredients and extracting the oil is the simplest and least expensive method.

Pressing the flowers into trays of fat and adding fresh blooms every day for up to three months until the fat is saturated with essential oil is the most labor- and time-intensive method. After pressing citrus fruit peel by hand or by machine, the oil is collected in sponges below. Typically, plant resins are combined with alcohol and a solvent to aid in the extraction of the gum resin's essential oil.

Assess Your Smell

We use our sense of smell less often now than in the past. Once, it showed us the way to food, alerted us to danger or adversaries, and led us to our friends' campfires. The majority of us have now compromised our sense of smell to the extent that we only detect odors that are overly pleasing or disagreeable. The nose ignores everything in between. Nevertheless, our mind nevertheless responds to certain odors. Just as freshly cut grass calms you down when you're agitated, freshly cooked meal makes you relax when you're hungry.

Aromatherapy, which has emerged as one of the most promising new fields of industrial research, is based on this innate reaction to smell. 'Mood' perfumes are being developed by perfume producers in France to improve both the wearer's mood and appearance simultaneously.

Air conditioning systems that release essential oils gradually and keep drivers attentive while operating a vehicle are currently the subject of research by American automakers. An alarm clock that releases scent ahead of time to help you wake up feeling nice is available in Japan. Additionally, hospital patients in the UK are given calming scents to help them get ready for therapy.

These kinds of advances will soon restore the importance of our sense of smell.

The human nose can detect over 10,000 distinct scents, but since we've grown so indolent, most of us are only able to identify a tenth of them. Fortunately, just like a lot of other things, fragrances can be remembered and relearned. All you need to do is teach your nose to recognize the various scents it comes into contact with.

Here are two easy tests to help you with that: (1) find out how good your sense of smell is; and (2) find out which essential oils you would like best. Both tests involve ordinary home materials.

You can take the first test alone; the second requires you to wear a blindfold and have a buddy or partner help you.

1. ***The Sniff And Guess Test:*** Have your companion select ten items from your home inventory using the table provided at the conclusion of this chapter. Don your blindfold and refrain from snooping; it's crucial that you are unaware of the people who have been chosen. To guess what the object is, your companion must cut any fruit, smash fresh (not dried) herbs, and open jars, bottles, or tubes. They must then hold each item, one at a time, around three inches from your nose tip for up to thirty seconds. You have an above-average sense of smell if you correctly answer five or more

questions. Don't, however, get complacent. Practice until you achieve a score of ten out of ten.

2. ***The Scent Family Test:*** Once more, select three products from each group (three floral, three citrus, three green, etc.) using the chart at the conclusion of this chapter. Place the ones you like on one side and the ones you don't like on another, then mix them around and smell them at random. It helps if you keep your eyes closed while you sniff, as this will help you to concentrate on the smell rather than what you see. Next, determine which fragrance categories you were most fond of. These are the groups that you are inherently drawn to. You might like citrus and green flavors, for instance, over floral, woodsy, and spicy ones. The section "Best Oils to Buy" lists the most popular essential oils under each category of fragrance. When you first start purchasing oils, limit your selection to the categories you naturally gravitate toward. Most reputable providers have at least 40 oils.

Best Oils To Buy

When purchasing essential oils, the most important guideline is to follow your nose. Smell is a profoundly personal sense, connected as it is to our memories and emotions associated with certain fragrances. While eucalyptus may bring back memories of an Australian vacation for your closest friend, it only makes you feel afraid, just like when you were a child in the hospital with pneumonia.

Don't try to smell every oil in the store on your first shopping excursion. There are so many that you will simply become perplexed. Make a note of the 10 oils that most interest you from a therapeutic standpoint and begin by sniffing those. The human nose is easily fatigued and shuts down when it is overstimulated.

Trusted Mixers

Generally speaking, oils that blend well with the greatest number of other oils are the most beneficial. They must also have the most pleasing scents along with the widest range of therapeutic applications. This is the perfect little assortment:

Start with	Handy Extras
Jasmine	Chamomile
Lavender	Eucalyptus
Neroli	Geranium
Peppermint	Lemon
Rose	Patchouli
Sandalwood	Ylang-Ylang

The Groups of Fragrance

Determining which aroma categories you naturally prefer is another approach to cut down on the quantity of essential oils you originally select. Use the sniff-tests mentioned above to find out. Green, spicy, floral, citrus, and balsamic/woody are the five primary categories. None of them are to everyone's liking. Once you've determined what you like, focus on the essential oils that fit into those categories and add them to your collection first.

Green	Spicy	Floral	Citrus	Woody/ Balsamic
Basil	Cinnamon	Face Cream	Disinfectant	Aftershave
Clary Sage	Cloves	Honey	Lemon	Burnt Toast
Celery	Coriander	Honeysuckle	Lime	Coffee
Majoram	Gin	Jasmine	Marmalade	Leather
Melon	Ginger	Lavender	Orange	Peanut Butter
Mint	Mustard	Lilies	Tangerine	Pencil Shavings
Rosemary	Nutmeg	Peach		Tea
Thyme	Peppercorn	Perfume		Vinegar
Toothpaste	Sherry	Roses		Wax Polish
White Wine				

Chapter 1: Using Essential Oils

With their delightful scents and magical compounds that enhance health and well-being, essential oils are a joy to use in a variety of ways around the house. Furthermore, they don't require any elaborate preparation or specialized tools, regardless of how you utilize them. Breathing in and unscrewing the bottle can be all that is required.

Here are some ideas for the best ways to use essential oils to demonstrate the significant impact they can have on your life.

Air Purifier

Adding your favorite essential oil to your vacuum cleaner's dust bag is one of the simplest methods to smell your entire home (see chapter "Inhaling Essential Oils"). The oil will fragrance the room you are cleaning as the air is blown out. If you would like to utilize different scents on a regular basis, place the oil drops on a cotton ball next to your cleaner's internal exit filter. This facilitates switching up scents.

Baths

The most calming application of essential oils is in a bath. To reap the full advantages, all you need to do is a few drops of oil (see chapter "Essential Oils In Bath") in a hot water tub. The two primary ones are water to soften skin and hasten the absorption of oil, and steam and warmth to evaporate the oils and heighten the perfume. All you need to do is take a 15-minute nap while lying back.

Beauty Treatments

Certain essential oils are excellent for relieving skin irritation, while others promote rapid skin healing, revitalize aging skin, minimize oil production, or simply smell amazing applied to the face. They provide amazing beauty treatments, such as cleansers, masks, facials, and moisturizers (see chapter "Essential Oils for the Face"), that instantly improve your appearance and well-being.

Bedtime Treatments

Before you go to bed, put a few drops of your favorite oil on a tissue and place it next to your pillow so you may breathe it in as you sleep (see chapter "Inhaling Essential Oils"). You can use aphrodisiac oils, oils for relaxation, oils for headaches, colds, and sleeplessness, and oils to improve moods or confidence. Apply on a handkerchief for use during the day, as the scent lasts longer on fabric.

Body Moisturisers

Since essential oils penetrate skin so quickly and deeply, they are a great, affordable, and luxurious way to moisturize your body (see Chapter "Essential Oils for the Body"). Add them to a rich carrier oil, such apricot, jojoba, or peach, and blend them in any way for their aroma, therapeutic action, or both. Alternatively, just tack on a few drops of essential oil to the least expensive, most basic body moisturizing lotion available.

Cold Compresses

Use them to lower fever and calm inflammation (see the chapter on "Inhaling Essential Oils"). The process is the same as for poultices; however, use ice-cold water instead of hot.

Deodorisers

Essential oils for deodorization (refer to the chapter on "Inhaling Essential Oils") effectively eradicate germs and viruses. Burning oils in a vaporizer will sterilize the air in a sickroom. To stop odors, rub a few drops over the insoles of your shoes or leave a few drops on a cotton ball inside your laundry basket and closet.

You can obtain the same effect with a few droplets land on the inside underarm seam of shirts or sweaters.

Footbaths

Put a few drops of essential oil (see chapter "Essential Oils for the Bath") in a basin of water, then take a seat and soak your toes for the most luxurious footbath. You can add oils just for fragrance, or oils that assist relieve aches, stimulate circulation in chilly feet, revitalize weary feet, or lessen sweating.

Hair Care

Certain essential oils are quite effective for treating lifeless, thinning, or dull hair (see the chapter "Essential Oils for Common Problems"). You can saturate a moderate, fragrance-free shampoo with a few drops of oil. Alternatively, combine it with olive oil and apply a weekly deep conditioning massage to the scalp.

Hot Poultices

See the chapter on "Inhaling Essential Oils" for the best method of using essential oils to ease chest congestion and relieve muscle pain. In a bowl of boiling water, add a few drops of essential oil. Then, with rubber gloves on, submerge the cloth in folded cotton or flannel. After that, drain any extra water, cover the affected region, and wait for it to cool down to body temperature. Repeat the procedure after reheating.

Household Cleansers

As you'll learn in the chapter "Inhaling Essential Oils," some of the most antibacterial essential oils also work wonders as natural household cleaners. Use a moist cloth to dab at work surfaces or trash cans after adding a few drops to it. Alternately, mix with a bucket of warm water to clean kitchens, bathrooms, and floors. They are less priced, non-chemical, and smell better than the majority of store-bought cleansers.

Inhalation

One of the finest ways to treat colds or coughs is to inhale essential oils. In a bowl of boiling water, add a few drops of oil, cover your head with a towel, bend over the bowl, and take long, deep breaths for a few minutes. In order to deep-cleanse, moisturize, or brighten a dull complexion, steaming is an excellent way to enjoy a facial (see chapter "Essential Oils for the Face"). Steam also opens pores and allows oils to penetrate the skin.

Insect Repellent

Certain essential oils have strong natural insecticidal properties (see the part on "Inhaling Essential Oils"). A moist cloth should be dampened with a few drops of essential oil, then used to wipe out interior wardrobes, the area around window frames, or the hems of drapes.

Massage

The most popular application for essential oils is massage (refer to the chapter "Using essential oils for massage"). Combining the senses of touch and smell, some would argue that it is the most enjoyable. Because essential oils are diluted in a carrier oil, such as sunflower, and applied directly to the skin, it is also the most therapeutic approach. Two additional benefits of massage are that it increases circulation, which allows the oils to spread quickly throughout the body, and it intensifies the scent of the oils due to the heat generated by the skin-on-skin friction, which expedites the body's and mind's healing effects.

Pot-Pourri

To create your own potpourri, combine a bowl of dried flowers, herbs, grasses, or seed pods with a few drops (refer to the chapter "Inhaling Essential Oils") of a broad blend of floral, spicy, and citrus essential oils. After a brief period of time, cover the bowl and let the smells seep in. Next, toss in the dried flowers and mix to ensure they absorb the flavor. Your room will smell like potpourri for up to six weeks.

Room Sprays

Using your personal favorite scents, combine a few drops of essential oil with water in a pump-action spray container to create a therapeutic air freshener (see chapter "Inhaling Essential Oils"). Thoroughly shake before using.

Room Vaporisers

These offer a method of preheating essential oils so that their scents swiftly fill the space (refer to the chapter on "Inhaling Essential Oils"). Vaporisers are little pots with a saucer-shaped top that holds water supplemented with a few drops of essential oil and a bowl-shaped bottom that holds a candle. The water is heated by the flame, and the oil quickly vaporizes and spreads throughout the atmosphere. Placing a saucer of warm water on top of a hot radiator and a few drops of oil in the water will have the same effect. Ring burners can also be purchased. They sit around a lightbulb, which heats the liquid and releases the essential oil's scent, and they hold a few drops of essential oil.

Wood Fires

About fifteen minutes before starting the fire, add a few drops of your favorite essential oil to the wood (see the chapter on "Inhaling Essential Oils"). The aroma will fill the room as a result of the heat. This is especially delicious with something special like oranges, ginger, and sandalwood around Christmas and other family gatherings.

As you may have already realized, I will go into great detail about each of these applications in the upcoming chapters so you can fully comprehend them and learn how to use them in your day-to-day activities.

Chapter 2: How to Use Essential Oils

Because essential oils are highly concentrated, they should never be used without first being diluted—either in water for a bath or with a simple carrier oil for a massage. Applying twice as much essential oil does not necessarily result in twice as many advantages because certain oils are extremely poisonous and others will make you feel queasy when used in excess. And they are all measured in drops because they are all so potent.

Always follow the directions for each specific recipe precisely to ensure that you are using essential oils correctly, safely, and to their fullest potential. Make care to read the cautionary list located later in this chapter. Because essential oils can be highly costly (one gram of jasmine, for example, can cost almost as much as one gram of gold), it's important to dilute, blend, and store them properly to extend their shelf life without sacrificing quality.

How To Dilute Essential Oils

There is always a drop quantity for essential oils. The majority of the tiny, 10-ml (12 fluid ounce) black glass bottles in which they are often offered have droppers integrated into the caps. If not, though, you can measure out droplets with a pipette or eyedropper. If you are using multiple oils, make sure to completely wash the dropper between each one to avoid blending the oils and destroying their distinct scents.

Because essential oils are so evaporative, it's important to measure out drops precisely and promptly. Should you unintentionally spill the bottle, wipe it up right away with paper towels, tissue, or a toilet roll before giving it a warm water and detergent wash. If you simply leave the oil on the surface, it will evaporate throughout the space and, if it's too strong, can give you the flu or headaches.

This book's recipes show for precise drops of essential oils. However, if you are creating your own mixtures, you can apply the following general guidelines for safe dilution:

For Massage

- 15-20 drops essential oil in 60ml (2 fl oz/12 tsp) carrier oil

- 7-10 drops essential oil in 30ml (1 fl oz/6 tsp) carrier oil

- 3-5 drops essential oil in 15ml (1/2 fl oz/3 tsp) carrier oil

For Bath

- 8-10 drops maximum essential oils in any one bath

How To Blend Essential Oils

Prior to being massaged or applied anyplace on the skin, essential oils need to be combined with a base or carrier oil. You can use any pure, cold-pressed plant oil since it helps disperse the essential oils uniformly, slows down their rate of evaporation, and increases their absorption into the skin. It also dilutes the essential oils to make them safe.

When combining essential oils, measure out the carrier oil beforehand and store it in a glass bottle if storing it or a ceramic bowl if using right away. After that, incorporate the essential oil drops thoroughly. Make sure to clearly label the bottle with the amount of essential oil drops in the mixture if you are producing enough for future usage.

Selecting a high-quality, pure vegetable oil to use as a carrier for your essential oils is crucial. Due to its low penetration capabilities, mineral oil, sometimes commonly referred to as baby oil, is not a good carrier.

Best Carrier Oils For Body	Best Carrier Oils For Face
Grapeseed	Apricot Kernel
Peanut	Avocado
Safflower	Evening Primrose (for wrinkles)
Sesame (for stretch marks)	Jojoba
Soya	Peach Kernel

Best Carrier Oils For Body	Best Carrier Oils For Face
Sunflower	Sweet Almond
Sweet Almond	

How To Store Essential Oils

Pure essential oils should be kept out of direct sunlight, out of children's reach, in dark glass, airtight bottles, and in a cool environment. In this manner, they need to remain flawless for as long as a year.

Essential oils can be stored for up to six months after being diluted with a carrier oil and supplemented with one teaspoon of wheatgerm oil or the contents of a vitamin E capsule. This preserves your combination and functions as an antioxidant. If not, refrigerate it to prevent rancidity of the carrier oil. To keep oils as effective and fresh as possible, it is always better to blend them in little amounts for aromatherapy.

How To Combine Essential Oils

The fundamental guideline for making your own essential oil formulations, whether for therapeutic or recreational purposes, is to start out simple and work your way up to more complex ones.

Certain essential oils balance each other out, while others work against each other. In a medicinal sense, others support one another. For instance, lavender enhances the anti-inflammatory properties of chamomile. And some complement everything, particularly rose and lavender.

10 Best Mixers
Bergamot
Chamomile
Frankincense
Geranium
Jasmine
Lavender
Neroli
Rose
Sandalwood
Ylang-ylang

Learning How To Mix

See section "Best Oils To Buy" for a quick reference on which oils go well together when you first start putting your own combinations together. Also keep in mind that less is more. For the majority of blends, use just three oils per blend. Sometimes you can use four, but only if they belong to the same scent group (see the table at the end of the "Introduction" chapter). For example, you could use four essential oils that are flowery, like neroli, rose, lavender, and ylang-ylang.

Try your mixture before mixing it to avoid wasting essential oils. Cutting up some large strips of blotting paper is the best way. If using equal amounts of oils, apply one drop of each oil to the tip of one blotter strip. Put two drops of the oil that will predominate your recipe above the others onto the blotter's tip. Next, while inhaling, fan the greasy tips forward and backward beneath your nose while holding the strips together by their lower ends.

Follow your nose to determine whether the combination appeals to you, and blend it. Aromatherapy is particularly personal since our favorite scents are as much a result of the memories and emotions they arouse as from their actual smell. While you could love a combination you are creating for someone else, make sure you test it out on them first using blotting paper.

Male Favourites	Female Favourites
Basil	Bergamot
Bergamot	Geranium
Eucalyptus	Jasmine
Frankincense	Lavender
Jasmine	Neroli
Lavender	Patchouli

Male Favourites	Female Favourites
Lemon	Peppermint
Patchouli	Rose
Pine	Sage
Sandalwood	Ylang-ylang

Essential Equipment

- Large, dark glass, stoppered bottles for storing combinations of oils

- A ceramic bowl for immediate use

- A small funnel for pouring carrier oils into bottles

- Four eye-droppers/pipettes (You can start with one if you wash it thoroughly after each use, but with four it's a lot easier)

- 10-ml (12-fluid-oz) dark glass bottles with stoppered caps for storing pure essential oils

- Strips of blotting paper

IMPORTANT: Never use metal containers or bowls.

Oils To Use With Moderation	Oils To Avoid In Pregnancy	Photo-Toxic Oils
Basil	Angelica	Angelica
Bay	Basil	Bergamot
Camphor	Cedarwood	Citronella
Fennel	Citronella	Ginger
Ginger	Fennel	Lemon
Laurel	Juniper	Lime
Sage	Laurel	Mandarin
Tarragon	Marjoram	
Thyme	Myrrh	
Valerian	Rosemary	
	Sage	
	Tarragon	
	Thyme	
	Yarrow	

Always Follow Cautionary Instructions

Essential oils may do wonders for your mood, behavior, mental and physical health, and sense of smell, to name just a few. If you utilize them correctly, using them is also a terrific pleasure. These are the fundamental guidelines to make sure you won't run into any issues.

- Because essential oils are powerful, you should only ever measure them in drops.

- With the exception of lavender for small wounds and burns and tea tree for spots, fungal infections, etc., never apply undiluted essential oils to skin. Even these two should only be used moderately.

- Avoid ingesting essential oils. Oral therapy can only be prescribed by a licensed aromatherapist; otherwise, it is risky.

- The efficacy of essential oils is not increased by increasing their dosage. Certain oils are, in fact, harmful in excess.

- Keep essential oils away from children's reach. If any spills get into an eye, clean it out with a few drops of sweet, pure almond oil instead of water and get medical help.

- After a massage with essential oils, wait two hours before taking a bath or shower. Certain oils require that much time to completely permeate skin.

- Because glass bottles are particularly slippery to grip, it is better to avoid using them for essential oils massage mixes if you have greasy hands. Instead, use a bowl and soak your hands in it.

- Pure or diluted essential oils shouldn't be kept in plastic storage containers since this could lead to contamination.

- Use essential oils therapeutically to cure common ailments, but only as directed by a physician if symptoms don't go away.

- After applying citrus oil, avoid exposing your skin to the sun for six hours. They become phototoxic and might irritate skin after being exposed to the sun.

Chapter 3: Inhaling Essential Oils

Inhaling essential oils is one of the greatest ways to use them.

An essential oil's aroma has a variety of effects on you as you breathe it in.

First of all, the smell is immediately registered in the limbic region of the brain, which is also where memories and feelings are stored. Because of this, if your experience with antiseptics is associated with being in a hospital, the smell of an antiseptic may cause you to get scared. Alternatively, if your grandma used lavender as a perfume, the scent can remind you of a warm and safe embrace. This explains why you have such a strong sense of smell and why you either love or dislike a certain scent.

Second, each essential oil molecule is made up of tiny chemical components that are absorbed by the nasal membranes. These components can have a variety of effects, such as modifying mood, relaxing the nervous system, or increasing alertness. Researchers have physical evidence that this occurs, even if they are still unsure of how it does. For instance, they are aware that breathing in a calming scent instantly lowers blood pressure and reduces the pulse rate.

Both of these indicate that a quick, easy, and efficient way to benefit from essential oils' therapeutic properties is to inhale them. Aromatherapy is a great way to enhance your health and well-being and test and strengthen your sense of smell if you use it regularly. Additionally, everyone who enters your house will gain something.

The following part of this chapter contains some of the best essential oil combinations for each method, along with instructions on how to produce and use essential oils for inhalation.

Inhalation

When inhaling the oils in a confined space with warm steam, you obtain the most advantages in the shortest amount of time. It is perfect for giving your skin a steam facial (see chapter "Essential Oils for the Face") or for treating colds and coughs.

The best way is to put one liter (two pints) of boiling water in a basin that can hold heat and then top it over with five drops of essential oil. To capture the steam and evaporating oils, bend forward over the bowl and cover your head with a wide cloth. After breathing in the fumes for a few minutes, add a little more boiling water to remove any last traces of essential oil.

Undiluted essential oils can also be inhaled, but only sparingly, through a tissue or handkerchief. It will last for several hours if two drops of oil are applied straight onto the fabric. At night, place it on your pillow; during the day, put it in your bra or breast pocket.

Best Oils For Inhalation	Benefits
Chamomile	For insomnia or difficulty to fall asleep
Eucalyptus	For nasal or chest congestion and in general for respiratory health
Frankincense	For anxiety or depression
Myrrh	For cough or sore throat
Peppermint	For improving concentration and energy

Pot-Pourri

Create a DIY potpourri by combining dried leaves, dried flowers, and dried herbs from your garden (such as geranium, rose, lavender, pinks, cornflowers, and citrus blooms), along with some talcum powder, your favorite essential oils, and spices like cinnamon sticks, cloves, nutmeg, and allspice. Twelve drops of essential oil, two teaspoons of talc, and six cups of dry botanicals should make form the basic mixture.

Once the talc and dried materials have absorbed the smells, leave it in an airtight container and shake and invert it every day for a period of two weeks. Then, to scent a space, put it in an open bowl or jar. When necessary, refresh it with a few additional drops of aromatic oils.

Room Sprays

Ten drops of essential oil added to half a litre (one pint) of water in a pump-action spray bottle (the kind used for watering houseplants) will create a natural, non-aerosol, very scented air freshener. Before releasing four or five sprays into the air to freshen, deodorize, and perfume a room, give the mixture a thorough shake.

Best Oils For Room Sprays	Benefits
Lavender	To kill airborne germs in your home
Lemon	To refresh air in your toilet
Peppermint	To remove the stale smell of cigarette smoke

Best Uses & Combinations

Quantity	Oils	Benefits
5 drops each	Lemon & Lime	Deodorising the house from cooking smell and also wardrobes, cupboards and bathrooms
3 drops each	Lavender, Pine & Rosemary	Disinfecting damp or mould and also trash cans and bathrooms

Room Vaporisers

Essential oil burners with a saucer positioned over a candle stand are available for purchase. To keep the water hot enough for the essential oil to evaporate, fill the saucer with hot water, add up to eight drops of oil, and light the candle. They merely need to be put on a stable, secure surface that is out of children's and pets' reach in order for them to scent a space swiftly. Replace the oil and water every three to four hours.

A homemade version can be achieved by placing a saucer filled with hot water over a radiator that receives central heating; however, the oils do not evaporate as quickly as they would with a candle's heat.

Additionally, you may purchase little compressed card or metal rings that fit over a regular lightbulb to softly warm the four or five essential oil drops that are placed on them. They fragrance a space almost as rapidly and strongly as burners do.

Nebulizers, or electronic diffusers, are helpful because they allow essential oils to be utilized without being heated and therefore changed.

Combinations of multiple essential oils don't preserve each one's unique scents very well, so it's recommended to use only one essential oil at a time to smell a space. There is lots of diversity, though, as you may switch up the oils every day if you'd like.

Best Oils For Room Vaporisers	Benefits
Bergamot	Deodorizing, uplifting & refreshing
Eucalyptus	Mental alertness & unblocking nose or chest congestion
Geranium	Energizing yet relaxing
Jasmine	Boosts self-confidence & euphoria (Ideal during dinners & parties)
Lavender	Helps tiredness, tension & nerves
Mandarin	Soothing & calming, helps insomnia
Neroli	Sensual, soothing & calming
Peppermint	Boosts alertness & energy
Sandalwood	Romantic, relaxing & mellowing
Ylang-ylang	Sensual, Hypnotic & uplifting

Wood Fires

Pour up to 12 drops of essential oil onto three pieces of wood approximately 15 minutes before starting a fire, as heat increases the potency of essential oils. It will simultaneously smell and warm your space. You can get a similar effect by putting your favorite essence on a radiator if you don't have an open fire.

50

Best Oils For Wood Fires
Geranium
Jasmine
Lavender
Lemon
Lime
Neroli
Orange
Patchouli
Rose
Sandalwood

Best Combinations

Season	Quantity	Oils
Summer	4 drops each	Lavender, Geranium & Bergamot
Winter	4 drops each	Sandalwood, Ginger & Orange

Using Oils Around Your Home

There are more benefits to using essential oils in your home than just eliminating odors and irrational rage. Compared to many household cleansers, oils have stronger disinfection qualities that fight germs and enhance cleanliness. Another benefit is that the oils are truly natural and don't require any chemical additives that harm the environment in order to function as cleaners.

You only need a few drops of essential oil for most cleaning tasks, making them incredibly affordable and long-lasting. Additionally, there are situations where using the least amount of oils feasible is preferable so that they disinfect without giving off an overpowering scent.

Here are some ideas for using oils to protect, clean, and purify your house, along with recommendations for the best oils for the purpose.

Best Household Oils
Bergamot
Cedarwood
Eucalyptus
Geranium
Lavender
Lime
Mandarin
Myrrh
Orange
Peppermint
Pine
Sandalwood

Air Purifier

By adding essential oils to your vacuum cleaner's dust bag, you can not only create a fresh scent throughout your entire home but also improve air quality. Five drops of oil should be placed on a cotton-wool ball within the cleaner, up near the exit filter where the machine's air is released. To alter or renew the scent, simply swap it out for a fresh cotton ball as needed.

Best Oils For Purifying Air
Bergamot
Citronella
Lavender
Lemon
Peppermint
Pine
Rosemary
Tea-Tree

Cleansers

In a small bucket of warm water, add eight drops of essential oil and wring out a cloth to clean floors, kitchen surfaces, and chopping boards.

Use a moist towel and three drops of essential oil to clean sinks, toilets, and basins.

Two drops of essential oil should be added to the dishwashing water to disinfect dishes and utensils.

Three drops of essential oil should be added to the last rinse water when washing garments.

Best Oils For Cleaning	Best Use
Geranium & lavender mixed	For washing up
Lemon & lavender mixed	For basins, baths, sinks
Lemon & geranium mixed	For surfaces, like kitchen, etc
Tea-tree or pine	For toilets

Deodorisers

Utilize a vaporizer and burn oils as previously mentioned to purify the air in a sickroom.

Put four drops of essential oil on a cotton ball and store it in a closet, laundry basket, trash can, shoe rack, etc. to neutralize and deodorize odors.

Put two drops of essential oil within the underarm seams of shirts, jackets, or jumpers to address lingering underarm odor.

Use a tissue to massage four drops of essential oil into the insoles of odorous shoes.

Best Oils For Deodorising

For A Sickroom	To Neutralise Odours	For Underarm Odour	For Smelly Shoes
Eucalyptus (For Congestion, Colds)	Bergamot	Bergamot	Lemon
Tea-Tree (For Viruses, 'Flu, Etc)	Lavender	Citronella	
Lavender (Antiseptic, Calming, Relaxing)	Lemongrass		
Myrrh (Sore Throat, Coughs)	Peppermint		
Bergamot (Deodorising, Uplifting)	Thyme		

Insect Repellent

Essential oils are a great source of natural, scented, non-toxic pesticides that are repellent to insects yet kind to people. In a pump-action spray bottle, combine 15 drops of essential oil with 100ml (20fl oz/1 pint) of water. Shake well and then spritz into the air to frighten flying insects. Alternatively, apply five drops of essential oil to a moist towel and use it to clean the frames of doors, windows, shelves, and wardrobes. Alternatively, to ward off any aerial intruders, dab oil drops straight onto curtain hems.

With a few of drops of oil on your mattress or pillowcase, I can ward off pesky mosquitoes. As an alternative, before going to bed, dilute six drops of the essential oil in 30ml (1fl oz/6 tsp) sunflower oil and apply it onto any exposed skin. Additionally, it will lessen the itching from any insect bites.

Best Insect Repellent Oils	Use
Camphor	Moths
Citronella	Mosquitoes
Lemongrass	Most Flying Insects
Tea-Tree	Ants, Fleas, Most Insects
Thyme	Most Hopping/Crawling Insects

Special Remedies

To get rid of ants or cockroaches:
• Dilute eight drops of tea-tree and seven drops of thyme in 30ml (1fl oz/6 tsps) water in a spray bottle and spray everywhere they might walk.

To rid a pet of fleas:
• Dilute six drops of geranium, five drops of lavender and four drops of tea-tree in 30ml (1fl oz/6 tsps) of water in a spray bottle and spray into ruffled fur, carefully avoiding the eyes.

Poultices

This is the best method for applying essential oils to ease chest congestion and muscle soreness. Pour 100ml (20fl oz/1 pint) of extremely hot water into a saucepan, add five drops of essential oil, and cover. Take off the lid while wearing rubber gloves, then cover the water's surface with a folded piece of fabric or flannel to absorb oil. After removing any extra water, cover the affected region with it until it cools down to body temperature. Warm up again and do it again. Make sure a poultice isn't too hot by testing it first before applying it to skin.Hot packs can be applied to the following conditions: back pain, ear pain (apply one drop of oil to a moist cotton ball), cramps, boils, sore feet, arthritis, rheumatism, stomach ache, stiff neck, sore throat, or congestion in the chest.

Best Oils For Poultices

Aching Feet	Arthritis	Backache	Boils	Cramps	Earache
Citronella	Lime	Eucalyptus	Clary Sage	Ambrette	Lavender
Laurel	Myrrh	Lavender	Galbanum	Clary Sage	
Lemon	Spruce	Petitgrain	Lemongrass	Cypress	
Rosemary			Rosemary	Juniper,	
			Tea-Tree	Peppermint	
				Tarragon	

Muscular Pain	Rheumatism	Sore Throat & Congestion	Stiff Neck	Tummy Ache
Ambrette	Angelica	Angelica	Eucalyptus	Angelica
Basil	Lime	Eucalyptus	Spruce	Cypress
Bay	Pine	Ginger		Fennel
Camphor		Myrrh		Ginger
Eucalyptus		Peppermint		Peppermint
Ginger		Pine		Tarragon
Marjoram		Sandalwood		
Petitgrain		Thyme		
Pine				
Rosemary				

Cold Compresses

This is the best technique to use essential oils to lower fever or calm inflammation. Proceed as for the hot poultices, except submerge the oils in a bowl of 100ml (20 fl oz/1pt) cold water containing six ice cubes.

Use cold compresses for:

- Headaches
- Sprains
- Inflammation

- Fever

- Swollen Bumps

- Burns

- Blistered

- Sore Feet

- Rashes

- Measles

- Chicken Pox

- Sunburn

- Hangover

Best Oils For Cold Compresses

Blistered Sore Feet	Burns & Sunburn	Fever	Hangover	Headaches
Birch	Chamomile	Bergamot	Geranium	Basil
Geranium	Geranium	Tea-Tree	Neroli	Chamomile
Lavender	Lavender		Rose	Rose
Tea-Tree	Marigold			Violet
	Patchouli			

Inflammation	Measles & Chicken Pox	Rashes	Sprains	Swollen Bumps
Clary Sage	Bergamot	Cedarwood	Basil	Laurel
	Chamomile	Chamomile	Camphor	Rose
	Eucalyptus	Geranium	Citronella	
	Lavender	Marigold	Marjoram	
	Marigold	Violet		
	Tea-Tree	Yarrow		

Chapter 4: Using Essential Oils For Massage

Next method we are going to explore for applying aromatherapy in you life is the body massage with essential oils to help a variety of conditions.

One of the most popular applications for essential oils is massage, which is also how aromatherapists utilize them therapeutically. It provides immediate advantages for the body and mind since it integrates the sensations of touch and smell. The warm friction of the skin on the skin during a massage accelerates the absorption of essential oils and intensifies their aroma. Furthermore, the same friction improves blood flow, stimulates and relaxes muscles, decreases heart rate and blood pressure, and leaves you feeling better than you could have ever imagined.

Giving a massage using aromatherapy is quite easy. The primary guideline of any kind of massage is to trust your instincts, therefore you don't need to be an expert. You should feel your way over any lumps, tense or sore areas, and knotted muscles as you move your hands over the body. Employ basic strokes, but also trust your instincts and adjust the massage's pace, rhythm, and flow as you go. Continue using a certain stroke if the recipient appears to enjoy it; if they flinch, stop right away and try something new. Try the same motion with firmness, speed, and lightness.Get ready ahead of time. It won't be a soothing or enjoyable experience for either of you if you try to flip the pages of an open book alongside you with greasy fingertips. Read any directions before you begin.

Assemble everything you'll need, including the appropriate essential oils, in a warm, cozy space and then simply carry on from there.

How To Massage

Self-massage is the most effective technique to learn how to massage. Thus, four of the massages in this chapter—the anti-age facial, the energizing top-to-bottom, the relaxing foot, and the face/neck/scalp—can be performed by one person alone, but the final massage, the relaxing back, requires two hands. Even while giving yourself a massage is incredibly soothing, getting one from someone else is still more enjoyable. It's also very simple to modify the fundamental routines and perform them on someone else once you've mastered them on your own.

Basic Strokes

To warm the oils and facilitate their absorption into the skin, an essential oil massage requires a lot of long, slow strokes as well as brief, quick friction rubs. Apply greater pressure on the heavier muscles of the back, buttocks, and shoulders, and less pressure to the bony areas of the belly. The primary motions that you must learn to do are:

Stroking

This is the most basic massage technique: both hands are flat and the palms are down. You can stroke the cat-like object with one hand while moving the other behind it. or parallel motion in the same direction with both hands.

Raking

Assume that the tips of your fingers are a rake. Firmly pull them back towards you while keeping them bent but tight at the joints and your fingertips touching the skin. You have the option to utilize both hands simultaneously in this motion, or to alternately move one hand in front of the other.

Pummelling

Keeping your fingers loose and your hands clenched into fists, quickly bounce each one up and down on your body like a drum. You can perform it with your hands turned palm upwards, sideways, or flat (pumping with fingertips down, thumbs up, and little fingers down) (i.e. pummelling with backs of hands).

Friction Rub

Move one hand up and the other down in a quick, sawing motion, with the palms down and the hands flat.

Thumbing

Work into the flesh with the pad and side of your thumb, giving it thorough strokes. Additionally, you can press down, hold, and then release over deep muscle tissue using the tips of your thumbs, or you can use them to make small, deep circles.

Kneading

Lay your hands flat with your fingers together and your thumbs wide. Next, move your thumbs over the same piece of flesh, pinching and pushing the flesh up towards your fingers as you go.

What You Will Need

In addition to the proper essential oil, a warm, cozy space is necessary for an aromatherapy massage in order to ensure that the evaporating oils are as aromatic as possible and to prevent goosebumps. You need peace and quiet, so put the phone off the hook and switch off the TV.

Wear loose, easily removed clothing, and have plenty of large towels on hand to wrap about oneself or serve as pillows or cushioning. Blend a little amount of aromatherapy massage oil, and since oily hands make glass difficult to grip, transfer the mixture to a plastic bottle with a squirting top or a dish you can dip your fingers into.

The Basic Massage

Essential oils need to be diluted with a carrier oil before they are massaged into skin. The basic recipe should be:

For a body massage:

- 15 drops essential oil in 60ml (2fl oz/12 tsps) carrier oil

For a face or foot massage:

- 5 drops of essential oil in 30ml (1fl oz/6 tsps) carrier oil

To keep the essential ingredients fresh and uncontaminated, follow these recipes and mix only as much as needed each time. If you have more than you need, store any leftovers in a dark glass bottle with a tight stopper and keep it out of direct sunlight.

For every massage, you should use just enough oil to cause your hands to slip but not slide. Using little amounts of warm oil at first, apply it to your skin in rhythmic, flowing strokes, adding more to your hands when your fingers begin to drag over the skin.

The greatest carrier oils to provide sufficient slide for massage are safflower, sunflower, or sweet almond. These are great for the face and body, but choose one of the carrier oils made especially for facial skin care (see chapter "Best Oils for the Face") if you want to address a specific kind of skin condition or complexion as you massage.

When making your oils, measure the carrier first, then gradually add the essential oil drop by drop, shaking or stirring to combine. Generally speaking, you should only use three essential oils at a time when massaging; any more will merely cause the scents to clash rather than combine together.

How To Combine Oils

You can use one oil for massage, or you can combine two or three. The following list contains the top essential oils for a massage using just one aroma.

Best Aromatic Oils
Bergamot
Geranium
Lavender
Neroli
Orange
Rose
Ylang-Ylang

Best Therapeutic Oils	Benefits
Chamomile	Insomnia, Stress & Tension
Clary Sage	Pre-Menstrual Tension, Fatigue & Depression
Eucalyptus	Colds & Aching Muscles
Mimosa	Cheering & Anti-Depressant
Peppermint	Invigorating & Energising
Rosemary	Mental Fatigue & Headache
Sandalwood	Sensual, Sedative & Calming

The more fragrant the oils are while mixing them for a massage, the more sensuous the experience will be. When combined with the ideal scent to revive or replenish the body and mind, touch becomes even more calming. This implies that while many of the most therapeutic oils may be beneficial to you, a massage for pleasure also needs to smell good, thus they are not included in the following formulas. But if you're in need of a massage that's strictly therapeutic, consult the essential oil characteristics chart at the end of the book to help guide your selection.

Recall that to allow the essential oils in the massage to fully absorb, wait two hours before taking a bath or shower after receiving an aromatherapy massage. For each of the five massages in this chapter, here are some top picks for oils.

Relaxing Back Massage

One of the greatest parts of the body to massage is the back because of its complex network of muscles and nerves, which cause it to react strongly to light pressure. It's also a big, flat area that's perfect for practicing strokes and spreading oil.The top essential oils for aromatherapy are listed here.

Best Oils For Back Massage
Bergamot
Eucalyptus

Best Oils For Back Massage
Frankincense
Lavender
Orange
Petitgrain

Use	Best Combinations
Energising massage	6 drops bergamot, 5 drops peppermint and 2 drops of lemon in 60ml (2fl oz/12 tsps) sweet almond oil
For backache	6 drops each lavender and eucalyptus and 3 drops lemon in 60ml (2fl oz/12 tsps) safflower oil
For tense muscles	8 drops lavender, 5 drops petitgrain and 2 drops basil in 60ml (2fl oz/12 tsps) sunflower oil
Invigorating summer rub	6 drops orange, 5 drops lemongrass and 4 drops rosemary in 60ml (2fl oz/12 tsps) sweet almond oil
Relaxing massage	7 drops lavender and 4 drops each rose and mimosa in 60ml (2fl oz/12 tsps) sunflower oil
Warming winter rub	6 drops frankincense, 5 drops eucalyptus and 4 drops pine in 60ml (2fl oz/12 tsps) sunflower oil

Step-By-Step Back Massage

The most suitable position for a back massage is to lie face down on a firm mattress or well-padded floor, with a small cushion or rolled towel under your upper chest to support your head and neck. Keep the light low and the room warm. Warm your hands and the aromatherapy massage oil before starting by submerging the container in hot water for a few minutes. Use these instructions as a guide just for the least number of motions; the more times you repeat each stroke, the more soothing it becomes. Don't hesitate to add your own unique touches.

1. With your hands on your lower back, space them about two inches apart from the spine, with your palms flat. Move them up to the upper back, then out over the shoulders and back down to the beginning. Pushing up toward the heart with a light stroke downward is the heaviest stroke. Feel for any tight or sore points in the back with it while you warm and distribute the oil. For a somewhat deeper variant, spread your fingers wide on the upward stroke only, pressing in with your tips. Continue for a few minutes in a calming, consistent rhythm.

2. Gently slide your hands apart along the length of the back, with the palms flat halfway up the spine and the other between the shoulder blades. Repeat many times. Next, with your hands still in the starting position, move them diagonally across your chest until one ends on a hip and the other on the shoulder across from it. Repeat in both directions. To stretch and release muscles, each action should be one long, strong stroke. At the conclusion, hold the skin taut for a few seconds before releasing the tension.

3. Follow step 1 again, but as you reach the top, move your hands across the shoulders, bending your fingertips down to the collarbones. Pull the shoulder muscle at the base of the neck firmly back during the downward stroke. Repeat. With your fingers pointing down, place your hands beneath your hips and, working one hand at a time, pull upward from the side of your body toward your spine. Work your way up one side of the body, across the shoulders, and down the other side to the hip on the other side.

4. Placing your palms flat on either side of the spine above the waist, raise them to the neck, move them out over each shoulder, and then return to the starting position as you move to the upper back. Continue the stroke, then

71

make smaller circles around and over each shoulder blade with your fingertip instead of your palm. Next, massage the sides of the neck and upper back by placing your hands flat, fingers together, and thumbs open. As you work, move your hands to push flesh up to the fingers.

5. Repeat a few of the step 1 sweeping motions on the lower back. Next, position one thumb on either side of the spine, approximately an inch out. Using the thumb pads, gently press down for five counts, then release the tiny muscles that support the spine by relaxing. Continue doing this until you reach the top of the neck and the back. Start at the bottom and work your way up to the neck, making little circles with each thumb on either side of the spine. Finally, go over the same area with your fingertips, firmly moving up and down.

6. Now cover the entire back with the fluid, flowing strokes you learned in step 1. Next, move in a circular motion with your fingertips from the base of the back to the neck. Lastly, rake your fingers over the bend so that only the pads make contact again. Then, use quick, strong strokes to draw the pad in desired direction. In order to ensure that one hand follows the other in a continuous movement, begin raking at the neck and move down to

the hips. Reduce the pressure as you repeat a few times
to end with a light, leisurely movement.

The Head Massage

Anxiety, concern, focus, and overthinking all end up on the poor
old head and shoulders. In addition to relieving stiff, tight
muscles, a massage of the face, neck, and scalp delivers the
evaporating essential oils directly beneath your nose, where they
act most directly on an exhausted, stressed mind. The following
are a some of the top aromatherapy combos for the neck up:

Best Oils For Head Massage
Bergamot
Jasmine
Lavender
Neroli
Orange
Rose

Use	Best Combinations
Energising massage	3 drops bergamot and 1 drop each of geranium and peppermint in 30ml (1fl oz/6 tsps) sweet almond oil

Use	Best Combinations
For a hair tonic	3 drops lavender and 1 drop each rosemary and bay in 30ml (1fl oz/6 tsps) sweet almond oil
For a headache	2 drops each rose and lavender and 1 drop chamomile in 30ml (1fl oz/6 tsps) sunflower oil
For tense muscles	2 drops each petitgrain and lavender and 1 drop basil in 30ml (1fl oz/6 tsps) sweet almond oil
To go to sleep	3 drops sandalwood and 2 drops of chamomile in 30ml (1fl oz/6 tsps) sweet almond oil
Relaxing massage	3 drops each rose, geranium and lavender in 30ml (1fl oz/6 tsps) sweet almond oil

Step-By-Step Head Massage

A massage of the face, neck, and scalp can greatly relieve stiff or fatigued shoulders. To begin, choose a comfortable seat at a table facing an upright chair. You may choose to wrap a towel around your arms for warmth or wear an off-the-shoulder blouse. Ensure that your aromatherapy oil is readily available and at room temperature.

1. As you slowly bend your neck to one side until your ear is parallel to your shoulder, maintain a straight back. Feel the stretch tugging up the side of your neck as you hold it for five counts. After progressively straightening, repeat on the opposite side. Place your left hand, palm down, on top of your right arm while keeping your head up. Stroke forcefully down the side of the neck to the ear, then across the top of the shoulder. After 10 repetitions, switch hands and continue on the opposite side.

2. With the fingers extending down your back and the heel of your hand resting on your collarbone, bend your elbows and place your hands palm down over your shoulders on either side of your neck. Lower your head back while applying pressure to the shoulder muscle, pinching it between your fingers and palm. After 10 counts of holding, carefully raise your head and let go of your hands. Repeat. Drop your head, pinching into the shoulder muscle, first to the left and then, after five counts, to the right, all from the same starting position. Repeat.

3. As in step 2, bend your neck forward and reposition your fingertips over the shoulder muscles. Using strong fingertips, knead the muscle, working gradually up either side of the neck from the nape to the head. Next, trace

tiny circles with the first two fingers of each hand, starting at the top of the neck and moving down the base of the skull to each ear. Keeping your head bowed, lay your right hand palm down over the nape of your neck. Using one hand to follow the other, slowly and firmly lift upward from the nape to the crown of your head.

4. Using your fingertips, spread them from ear to ear along the hairline on top of your forehead. With your fingers stiff yet bent, gently press them into your scalp and move them in short, firm circles to cause the scalp to rotate. Inch by inch, return to the head's top gradually. Work your way up to the crown, starting at the nape of the neck. After that, quickly and firmly pull at small strands of hair near the roots between each thumb and index finger many times. To improve scalp relaxation and circulation, repeat over the entire head.

5. With your elbows resting on a table, bend forward. Lay the heel of each hand over one eye, letting go and inhaling deeply while you hold it for ten counts. Raise your right hand to a straight grip and lay the first three fingers across your forehead. From the nasal bridge, move carefully and firmly up between the brows to the hairline. Five times over, repeat. Press in softly and move from inner to outer brows with your first two fingers.

Five times over, repeat. Apply a strong, slow palm stroke from the ears to the forehead, temples, and hair with one hand on each side of the face. Repeat.

6. Make tiny circles all over the face, from the jaw, across the cheekbones, over the temples, down the hairline, and up to the middle of the forehead, using the tips of your first two fingers. Use a firm, slow palm stroke to repeat. Next, softly press into the curves of your face with your palms over your cheekbones and your fingers over your forehead. Hold this position for ten counts. Press in for ten counts, placing one palm across your forehead and the other across the back of your neck. Press in and hold with one hand over each ear on your head.

Energizing Body Rub

A daily top-to-bottom wake-up massage—which will soon be detailed step-by-step—brings blossoms to the overworked, overstressed, underexecuted body. Not only does it leave you feeling energized and ready to go, but it also relieves early morning aches and pains, cellulite, and tense muscles. The greatest oils that enhance stimulation overall are:

Best Oils For Energising Body Rub
Bergamot
Lavender
Lemon
Orange
Peppermint
Petitgrain

Use	Best Combinations
Energising massage	5 drops each petitgrain, orange and bergamot in 60ml (2fl oz/12 tsps) sunflower oil
For cellulite	4 drops each rosemary and lemon and 9 drops geranium in 60ml (2fl oz/12 tsps) sweet almond oil
For mental alertness	6 drops bergamot and 4 drops peppermint in 60ml (2fl oz/12 tsps) sweet almond oil
For summer	6 drops lavender, 5 drops orange and 4 drops peppermint in 60ml (2fl oz/12 tsps) sweet almond oil
For tight muscles	5 drops pine, 7 drops lavender and 3 drops eucalyptus in 60ml (2fl oz/12 tsps) sweet almond oil
For winter	7 drops lavender and 4 drops each peppermint and myrrh in 60ml (2fl oz/12 tsps) sunflower oil

Step-By-Step Energizing Body Rub

Although it only takes 10 minutes in the morning, this massage has lifelong benefits. The only equipment needed for the first step is a chair or the side of a bed or bathtub to place your foot on. The entire sequence is performed standing up. Before you start, make sure you have an ample supply of aromatherapy massage oil on available.

1. With one foot elevated on a chair so that the knee is at a straight angle, perform firm upward palm strokes from the ankle to the knee with one hand trailing the other. Work on the sides, rear, and front of each leg. To stroke from the knee to the top, front, rear, and sides of the thigh, straighten your leg. Next, repeat the motion with your hands joined so that one is raking the front of the leg while the other is raking the rear. This time, use stiff, bent fingers to rake the legs in an upward stroke. Additionally, use the same stroke up each leg's side.

2. Shake your hands loosely at your sides, floppy from the elbow down, as you're shaking off water. Raise your arms straight over your head, then extend them out to the sides in a shoulder-parallel manner and down to your toes. With your left hand, wrap your fingers around the upper arm, palm down, and make one strong stroke

down the arm to the elbow, then up the forearm from the elbow to the wrist. Bend your right arm so that it is at your shoulder. Proceed with the stroke, pressing the thumb into the palm and encircling the hand's back with fingers all the way up to the fingertips. On both arms, repeat.

3. Your hands should be in relaxed fists, and you should bounce them off the flesh in a quick, drumming motion to smash the tops of the thighs and buttocks. Beginning on your right side, perform a waist stroke by placing your left hand over your waist and your right hand over your hip with your fingers pointing to your navel. fingers pointing rearward. From hip to rib, make forceful, rhythmic upward strokes with one hand after the other. After completing 20 strokes in total, switch to the other side of the waist. Lastly, move the same rhythmic motion from the crotch to the ribs up the abdomen.

4. With your thumbs below and your index fingers above the collarbone, place your hands atop each shoulder and press and squeeze the bone, moving from the shoulder inward toward the chest. Pinch and knead the muscle between each hand's fingertips and heel while keeping your palms down. Then, place one hand back over each shoulder top. Next, place one hand palm down across the

nape of the neck, pinching and massaging the neck muscles as you relax the head slightly backward.

5. Stretch and hold your shoulders by rounding them forwards (head down), rearward (head back), up toward your ears, and down (head straight) while keeping your arms by your sides. Ten counts should be held for each stretch before you release it. Move your shoulders forward and backward once more, but this time, extend your arms straight out to your shoulders. Next, give yourself a hard headshake, as though you were removing water from your hair. Apply pressure to your scalp in tiny circles using straight, stiff fingers, just like you would when shampooing your hair.

6. With loose, floppy hands, give them a vigorous shake as though you're brushing water off them while bending your arms at the elbows. Next, for a count of sixty, move your hands in a fluid, flowing motion, from your brows to your forehead and into your hair, with one hand trailing the other. Put your left hand palm down on your forehead and your right hand palm down over the nape of your neck to finish with a forceful head press. Inhale with both hands, then hold the position for 15 counts. Unwind and carry on.

The Foot Massage

Compared to other body parts, the feet are subjected to greater maltreatment. Give them a relaxing, light massage as a thank you to spread happiness throughout your body.

Best Oils For The Foot Massage
Citronella
Geranium
Lavender
Lemon
Peppermint
Rosemary

Use	Best Combinations
Aromatic massage	2 drops each lavender, rose and geranium in 30ml (1fl oz/6 tsps) sunflower oil
For aching feet	3 drops eucalyptus and 2 drops chamomile in 30ml (1fl oz/6 tsps) sunflower oil
For excessive sweating	5 drops lemongrass in 30ml (1fl oz/6 tsps) sunflower oil
For fungal infections	3 drops tea-tree and 2 drops of geranium in 30ml (1fl oz/6 tsps) sunflower oil

Use	Best Combinations
Refreshing massage	2 drops each citronella and peppermint and 1 drop lemon in 30ml (1fl oz/6 tsps) sunflower oil
Relaxing massage	3 drops lavender and 2 drops geranium in 30ml (1fl oz/6 tsps) sunflower oil

Step-By-Step Shooting Foot Massage

Your entire body will feel better after the foot massage, which comes with a rejuvenating soak in aromatherapy prior that will put a bounce back in your step. To conclude the massage, take a seat erect and comfortably supported by cushions. Then, spend 10 minutes lying flat with your feet raised above your head.

You can use solely therapeutic essential oils for the bath and more sensual ones for the stroking that follows, or you can use the same essential oils for the massage and foot bath. Take your time and do as many extra repetitions of each step as you can.

1. With a big bowl of hot water on the floor or a plastic basin, take a comfortable seat first. Ensure that your aromatherapy massage oil, towels, and essential oils are all readily available. Soak both feet in the bowl with four drops of essential oil for every four liters (one gallon) of water. After ten minutes, leave one foot in the basin and begin massaging the other while it's still damp to improve the way the essential oils absorb. To give a massage, sit with one leg crossed over the other such that the calf rests on the thigh of the other leg.

2. Using the palms of your hands, place them between the foot and quickly rub it with a lot of oil, sawing back and forth over the foot. Beginning behind the arch, place one hand across the top of the foot and the other under it. Next, raise your hands so your palms are sandwiched between your toes and instep, on either side of your ankle. Finally, give your heels a vigorous rub. This is a useful method for increasing blood flow, warming up chilly feet, and completely relaxing them.

3. Stretch your feet a number of times to release tendons and relieve sore muscles. For ten counts, hold each stretch. Point and flex your toes, then hold them up, down, and to the left, right, and left again. To rotate the ankle, continue pointing your toes and slowly form big

circles in the air. Once your foot is back on your opposing thigh, lay your hand palm down over your toes, encircling the sole with your fingers. Push your toes down slowly to extend and flex them while maintaining a straight foot (i.e., a 90-degree angle with your leg) and hold. Next, slowly bring them back in the direction of the foot.

4. While maintaining the same posture, quickly pinch the entire heel of your foot for several minutes using the tips of your thumb and index finger. Next, round the top of the foot with your fingers, placing your thumbs beneath the arch and across the sole. Make sequential, deep, flowing thumbstrokes from the heel to the instep along the foot's arch. Then, lightly knead the sole of the foot by using the thumbs to create little circles.

5. Take a few minutes to gently massage each toe, starting at the base and working your way up to the tip, using your thumb on top and your index finger underneath. After that, bend your thumb underneath and use it to make several deep strokes up the bottom of each toe by crossing your fingers around the tips of your toes and pushing firmly and slowly. Lastly, give your toes a quick friction rub to warm them up and improve blood flow.

6. Using your thumb, massage and rub the entire area surrounding the ankle bone. Then, compress the tendon at the rear of the heel with your thumb and index finger. Step 3's foot stretches should be repeated, but this time, while you point, flex, and circle your ankles, keep both hands around them. Use multiple full footstrokes to close. Put one hand palm down over the foot and the other palm up under it. Beginning at the toes, move your hands in tandem to pull firmly and slowly, following the curve of your foot all the way back up to your ankle.

The Anti-Wrinkle Massage

An aromatherapy massage addresses the skin itself while relieving the anxiety and anger that lead to frowns, thus removing the stress marks from your face. It also promotes cell turnover, lessens fine wrinkles, and dehydrates the skin.

Regenerating Oils

Certain essential oils, like lavender, have the ability to promote the production of new skin cells. This explains why they work so well to cure wounds like burns and to maintain skin that feels smooth to the touch and looks healthy.

Best Oils For Anti-Wrinkle Massage
Geranium
Lavender
Myrrh
Neroli
Orange
Rose

Use	Best Combinations
Young skin (under 40)	3 drops geranium and 2 drops orange in 30ml (1fl oz/6 tsps) sweet almond oil
Mature skin (over 40)	2 drops each neroli and lavender and 1 drop myrrh in 30ml (1fl oz/6 tsps) wheatgerm oil
For oily complexions	2 drops each geranium and lavender and 1 drop bergamot in 30ml (1fl oz/6 tsps) sunflower oil
For dry complexions	3 drops rose and 2 drops neroli in 30ml (1fl oz/6 tsps) apricot kernel oil
For winter	2 drops each myrrh and sandalwood in 30ml (1fl oz/6 tsps) wheatgerm oil
For summer	2 drops each rose and violet and 1 drop geranium in 30ml (1fl oz/6 tsps) sunflower oil

Step-By-Step Anti-Wrinkle Massage

Nobody loves to see wrinkles on their own face, even though they are a symbol of a life well lived. Aside from surgery, there are just two things that can help prevent wrinkles: ensuring that skin is properly moisturized and shielded from the sun. Since essential oils naturally bond with skin and are absorbed into the body, they perform the latter function better than any other product.

1. Slide fingers up the side of the face to the temples after placing the first two fingers of each hand under each earlobe and softly pressing for a count of six. After softly pressing in for a count of six, remove the pressure and use your fingertips to gently draw little circles over the temples. position your little fingers side by side on the nose bridge. Then, with the other fingers spread wide apart and rigid, position them along each brow, with the index fingers resting on the temples. Apply light pressure, hold it for six counts, then apply pressure once again and work your fingers up the brow into the hairline, lifting the skin as you go. Finally, apply light pressure in small circular motions into the scalp. repeat five times.

2. Bend your head back and keep it there for six counts, opening your eyes wide and raising your eyebrows to stretch your neck. With your head up, line up your index fingers on the nose bridge and move them up, one after the other, from the brows to the forehead. After every sixth stroke, carefully extend one finger down each brow and press three times into the temple. Repeat many times. Next, move one hand after the other, palm-side up the forehead and into the hair, using the flat of your hand.

3. Start with the outer corner of each index finger and work your way slowly down the undereye, pressing gently inward for three counts until you are pressing in on the tear ducts. There is hardly any pressure at all throughout. Repeat along the browbone on the upper eyelid. Instead of dragging or stretching the skin, press in, raise it, and then press it again. While you relax and count to twenty, place the heels of each palm over the eyes and softly push. Lastly, firmly close your eyes and hold there for five counts. Next, spread them apart and gently roll your eyes three times in slow circles.

4. Bend the head to one side, keep it there for 10 counts, then move it to the other side and hold it there to extend the neck. With your head straight, make a rhythmic,

flowing motion with the backs of your fingertips from the clavicle to the chin. Then, with your palms facing up, quickly drum across your entire jawline, from ear to ear, using the first three fingertips of each hand to make a light, outward flick beneath your chin. Pinch the jawbone gently from the chin to the earlobes with your thumbs and forefingers. Go back to the chin's center and repeat.

5. With a relaxed jaw and an open mouth, move your chin to the left and hold for five counts, then to the right and hold for an additional five. Apply pressure with the tips of your little fingers to the center of your lower lip, hold it for five counts, and then repeat the motion, progressively extending to the corners of your mouth, then across the upper lip to the middle of your nose. Apply another gentle stroke. To conclude, place your palm over your mouth and hold it there for ten counts.

6. To promote circulation and enhance the color of your cheeks, place the palms of your hands against the sides of your face and quickly, lightly rub upwards. Apply the same stroke again, but this time, slowly and firmly stretch upward. Lastly, place your palms over your face and hold them there for 20 counts.

Chapter 5: Essential Oils for the Face

What most women agree upon as the hallmark of great beauty is a healthy, radiant complexion. As a result, people spend more money on skincare than on any other cosmetics. As a result, thousands of potions for the face alone have been developed by the cosmetics industry, including cleansers, toners, moisturizers, exfoliators, masks, eye creams and gels, neck creams, anti-aging serums, and sun and pollution protection.

Really, all you need is the appropriate essential oil. They are capable of doing all of these tasks, and because of their diverse variety of qualities, they can do so in a way that best meets the requirements of your skin.

Making your own essential-oil beauty products allows you to control exactly what ingredients are included. They are also custom-blended, incredibly powerful, aromatically fragranced, and incredibly affordable because you won't be paying for beautiful packaging or costly advertising efforts.

The Best Products For Beauty

Essential oils can be used to create products for your entire beauty routine, including deep cleansing, exfoliating, toning, and anti-aging treatments for your face. Additionally, each product can be created to address a different skin type or issue, such as open pores, acne, or older, dry complexions.Because the insides of the mouth, nose, and eyes are sensitive areas and essential oils are strong, exercise caution while applying essential-oil cosmetic products in these areas.

Make sure you use essential oils to their full potential because they may cure mental and emotional issues just as effectively as physical ones. Use them sparingly. For example, on a stressful day, massage your dry skin with rose and lavender oils to soothe your complexion and ease your mental troubles. Alternatively, if you're exhausted after a long day, try geranium and neroli oils to uplift your mood and look good at the same time.

Certain essential oils are healthier for the delicate facial skin than others, even though all essential oils are absorbed by the skin more effectively than the contents of the majority of cosmetic face creams. Because face skin differs from body skin, this is the case. exposed to the elements, air pollution, and sunshine for the entire day. Therefore, compared to other oils, the calming, restorative, and revitalizing essential oils will have a far more obvious effect on facial skin. Here is a list of the best facial oils to assist you make your decision.

Best Aromatic Oils For The Face
Geranium
Jasmine
Lavender
Neroli
Rose
Violet
Ylang-Ylang

Best Therapeutic Oils For The Face	Benefits
Chamomile	Rashes & Itchiness
Juniper	Acne & Oiliness
Lemongrass	Open Pores
Mandarin	Scars & Slack Skin
Marigold	Over-Dry & Sensitive Skin
Mimosa	Dull Complexions
Orange	Wrinkles & Sallowness

Cleansers

Certain women prefer to use a cotton ball drenched in cream cleansing lotion, while others believe that their faces aren't clean until they've splashed them with water. Nevertheless, incorporating the advantages of essential oils is simple regardless of the regimen you choose. Additionally, essential oils deeply clean pores and address issues at the same time because they absorb into skin rapidly and readily.

The following are the top oils to use every day to gently wash and calm skin:

- Neroli for dry or mature skin

- Rose for normal or mixed skin

- Lavender(for oily or blemished skin

The Water & Soap Clean

For your last facial rinse, if you wash with soap and water, mix two drops of essential oil into a basin of warm water. After using your fingers to gently mix the oil droplets, splash and pat the water onto your face. If you have the time, let the water air dry on the skin instead of wiping it off with a towel, allowing the essential oils to remain as a film.

The Oil Clean

If you often wash your face and remove makeup with a light, oil-based lotion, try substituting it with 30 ml (1fl oz/6 tsps) of sweet almond oil mixed with three drops of essential oil. Before putting any of the mixture into the palm of your hand, shake it well in a dark glass bottle. If any lingering makeup remains, remove it by dipping a cotton-wool ball into the oil mixture and gently wiping across the skin. Otherwise, gently wipe it off with a damp cotton-wool pad and massage it in with your fingertips.

The Cream Clean

You can incorporate the aroma and health benefits of essential oils into your regular cosmetic product if you choose to wash your face with a cream cleanser. For every 50ml (1.7fl oz/10 tsps) of product in the container, add four drops of essential oil to the simplest, fragrance-free washing cream you can find. Using a sterilized spoon or spatula handle, mix the essential oil into the cleaner. Replace the cover and let it sit for three days. Before using the mixture, give it one stir every day. Apply and remove it in the same manner as before.

Nevertheless, discard the formulation if, over these three days, you observe any changes in its texture, such as it becoming lumpier, thinner, or thicker. Addition of additional components can sometimes cause the emulsion of a specific brand of cream to become unstable, which can ultimately result in bacterial contamination.

The True Clean

Use a mild essential oil exfoliant twice a week for skin that is genuinely polished and free of dead, flaky, and dull surface cells.

Blend 30ml (1fl oz/6 tsps) sweet almond oil with three drops essential oil. Gradually add equal parts finely powdered oatmeal and coarse desiccated coconut until you have a thick paste. Apply the paste to your damp skin in small circular motions, paying special attention to the areas around your chin, forehead, nose, and neck. After a few minutes, rinse it off with lukewarm water. After patting dry, moisturize right away.

The Cleanser For Trouble Spots

Using essential oils in the same way for your complete beauty routine will increase their effectiveness. For instance, add your favorite-smelling anti-grease essential oils to your cleanser, toner, and moisturizer to address the issue of a very oily skin. Then, to target specific skin trouble areas, you can intensify your treatment by utilizing certain oils in weekly exfoliators, masks, or steam facials.You can also combine an oily and dry face moisturizer, or use face masks or cleansers in the same way, applying each type only where needed. Your complexion will benefit more the more you focus on and treat each of your unique skin issues—something you can never afford to do with traditional cosmetic products.To tailor your cleansers, refer to the recommended facial moisturizing recipes found further on in this chapter and use those specific essential-oil blends to ensure that the different phases of your skincare regimen work in harmony with one another.

Moisturisers

Essential oil-based facial moisturizers allow you to build wonderfully customized skincare products. Essential oils are so fine and naturally affine to skin that they penetrate better than many ingredients found in more conventional face creams. You can mix small amounts so the ingredients are always fresh without wasting any; you can mix several combinations for different parts of your face and apply them just where needed.

When to Use Them

They should be used to thoroughly washed skin both morning and night, just like any moisturizer. For a nighttime treatment, you can, however, use a thicker carrier oil and more hydrating essential oils, and make the product lighter for summer than for winter. Applying a moisturiser in the morning for enjoyment and aromatherapy is a great idea, as some of the treatment essential-oil combinations might not smell as good as some of the single oils, such the orange-blossom-scented neroli. Save the treatment items for the evening.

How to Use Them

Applying a face moisturizer sparingly is the ideal technique. If applied excessively, extra oil can lead to blackheads and other problems with glossy, greasy skin. The best technique to ensure that the oils absorb is to massage them in, as the warmth of the skin against the skin and the rubbing motion accelerate absorption. Use your fingertips to gently smooth the moisturizer over your entire face for at least three minutes, moving in circles from the inner to the outer corners of your eyes and moving them upwards. Even better, apply the self-massage technique for your face once a day to assist relax and tone your skin (see the detailed section on anti-wrinkle massage in chapter "Using Essential Oils For Massage").

To ensure that there is no chance of contamination, always remember to combine just enough to last a few days. Before using your moisturizer, always shake it well and store it in an airtight, dark glass bottle. The perfect recipe is Regarding moisturizers for the face Add one tsp of wheatgerm oil or the contents of a vitamin E capsule to 30ml (1fl oz/6 tsps) of carrier oil and five drops of essential oil.

How to Blend Them

Essential oils, dilution-enhancing carrier oil, and either vitamin E or wheatgerm oil should be present in all face moisturizers. The latter serve as a natural preservative and give your skincare an additional treatment benefit because they are both potent antioxidants.

According to the most recent ideas on skin damage and aging, cells oxidize—a process akin to that of an apple rotting or a metal rusting—when exposed to external irritants such as sunshine, pollution, or cigarette smoke. Studies reveal that antioxidants prevent this deterioration and aid in making up for damage regularly inflicted by skin irritants.The finest antioxidants to help prevent skin aging are vitamins C, E, and A, which are currently found in the majority of cosmetic face creams.

Thus, you are adding an anti-aging component to every facial moisturizer you mix by adding wheatgerm, which has a high level of vitamin E, or pure vitamin E obtained by pricking a capsule with a pin and squeezing out the contents.Another benefit is that carrier oils, which are used to dilute essential oils, have high moisturizing properties on their own. Recall that a good moisturizer is made of oil on the skin's surface, not some unknown moisturizing agent.

The oil prevents the body's natural water from evaporating and releasing into the atmosphere.

Fine, light emollients are the ideal carrier oils for the face. Certain thicker oils are very nourishing and leave the skin on the face glossy for hours.

Moisturisers For Troubled Spots

Use the charts to examine the qualities of essential oils before creating your own formulations for skin moisturizers. Use the specified chart to ensure that the oils of your choice will blend nicely together. To make sure your nose is happy with the final aromatic combination, you can also attempt the blotting paper sniff test (see chapter "Introduction").

Best Carrier Oils For The Face	Benefits
Apricot Kernel	For Dry Skin
Avocado	For Oily & Blemished Skin
Evening Primrose	For Wrinkles
Jojoba	For Greasy & Irritated Skin
Peach Kernel	For Sensitive Skin
Sunflower	For Oily & Blemished Skin
Sweet Almond	For Normal & Mixed Skin
Wheatgerm	For Mature Skin

Rich Moisturisers

For mature skin

Remedy #1:

- 3 drops neroli and 2 drops galbanum in 30ml (1fl oz/6 tsps) wheatgerm oil

Remedy #2:

- 2 drops each rose and frankincense in 30ml (1fl oz/6 tsps) evening primrose oil plus 1 vitamin E capsule

For dry skin

Remedy #1:

- 2 drops violet and 3 drops rose in 30ml (1fl oz/6 tsps) apricot kernel oil plus 1 vitamin E capsule

Remedy #2:

- 2 drops each neroli, mimosa and rose in 30ml (1f6z/6 tsps) wheatgerm oil

For thread veins

Remedy #1:

- 3 drops rose and 2 drops chamomile in 30ml (1fl oz/6 tsps) peach oil plus 1 tsp wheatgerm oil

Remedy #2:

- 3 drops orange and 1 drop each lemon and lime in 30ml (1fl oz/6 tsps) peach oil plus 1 tsp wheatgerm oil

To treat rashes, itchiness

Remedy #1:

- 2 drops chamomile and 3 drops lavender in 20ml (11) oz/6 tsps) peach oil plus 1 vitamin E capsule

Remedy #2:

- 1 drop each marigold and yarrow and 3 drops of sandalwood in 30ml (1fl oz/6 tsps) jojoba oil plus 1 tsp wheatgerm oil

To firm skin

Remedy #1:

- 3 drops frankincense and 2 drops mandarin in 30ml (1fl oz/6 tsps) wheatgerm oil

Remedy #2:

- 2 drops each rose and lavender and 1 drop neroli in 30ml (1fl oz/6 tsps) wheatgerm oil

To improve texture

Remedy #1:

- 3 drops violet and 2 drops lemongrass in 30ml (1fl oz/6 tsps) evening primrose oil plus 1 vitamin E capsule

Remedy #2:

- 2 drops each sandalwood and geranium and 1 drop rose in 30ml (1fl oz/6 tsps) wheatgerm oil

For night time

- 2 drops each frankincense and myrrh in 30ml (1fl oz/6 taps) wheatgerm oil

Light Moisturisers

For oily skin

Remedy #1:

- 2 drops each juniper and cedarwood in 30ml (1fl oz/6 tsps) sunflower oil plus 1 vitamin E capsule

Remedy#2:

- 2 drops each geranium and lavender and 1 drop cypress in 30ml (1fl oz/6 tsps) of sunflower oil plus 1 vitamin E capsule

For combination skin

Remedy #1:

- 2 drops each lemongrass and rosemary in 30ml (1f oz/6 tsps) sweet almond oil plus 1 vitamin E capsule

Remedy #2:

- 1 drop petitgrain and 2 drops each rose and lavender in 30ml (1fl oz/6 tsps) sweet almond oil plus 1 vitamin E capsule

For sensitive skin

Remedy #1:

- 2 drops marigold and 3 drops rosemary in 30ml (1fl oz/6 tsps) peach oil plus 1 tsp wheatgerm oil

Remedy #2:

- 2 drops each chamomile and jasmine and 1 drop sandalwood in 30ml (1fl oz/6 tsps) jojoba oil plus 1 vitamin E capsule

To treat sallowness

Remedy #1:

- 3 drops orange and 2 drops rosemary in 30ml (1fl oz/6 tsps) jojoba oil plus 1 tsp wheatgerm oil

Remedy #2:

- 2 drops each lavender and ylang-ylang and 1 drop geranium in 30ml (1fl oz/6 tsps) sunflower oil plus 1 vitamin E capsule

To treat acne

Remedy #1:

- 3 drops bergamot and 2 drops chamomile in 30ml (1fl oz/6 tsps) sunflower oil plus 1 vitamin E capsule

Remedy #2:

- 2 drops each lavender and mint and 1 drop lemon in 30ml (1fl oz/6 tsps) sunflower oil plus 1 vitamin E capsule

To clear blackheads

Remedy #1:

- 2 drops each tea-tree and eucalyptus in 30ml (1fl oz/6 tsps) avocado oil plus 1 vitamin E capsule

Remedy #2:

- 2 drops each lavender and geranium and 1 drop lemon in 30ml (1fl oz/6 tsps) sunflower oil plus 1 vitamin E capsule

For day time

- 2 drops violet and 3 drops rose in 30ml (1fl oz/6 tsps) sweet almond oil plus 1 vitamin E capsule

Face Masks

It only takes five minutes to make your own essential oil face mask, and you'll end up with a really useful product that you can enjoy doing yourself with basic kitchen items. Another benefit is that you only need enough for one application, which eliminates waste and allows you to experiment with different combinations as much as you'd like. Additionally, by including the paste that draws attention to the skin or the mask ingredient, you assist keep the essential oils where they belong on the skin's surface, where they are absorbed and become even more useful rather than escaping into the air. For a deep facial treatment, the following oils work best to fix to the skin's surface:

- Frankincense: For Mature & Dry Skin

- Jasmine: For Normal & Mixed Skin

- Geranium: For Oily & Blemished Skin

When to Use Them

Face masks can be utilized as nourishing or cleansing treatments only on occasion to improve the appearance of your skin while you're under stress, sick, or experiencing hormonal or climatic changes. They overstimulate skin, causing it to become drier or oilier if you use them excessively.

It is recommended to apply a moisturizing pack no more than twice a week and a deep-cleansing face mask no more than once. Using them at night is ideal, and since you will need to lie down and relax while the mask works, you can add an energizing or soothing fragrant oil to the mixture to help with your mental state as well.

How to Use Them

Once your essential oil face mask is ready, distribute it evenly over your cleansed skin using upward strokes. Apply the cream to the neck down to the collarbone, avoiding the eye region, lips, and nostrils because the skin in these areas is extremely sensitive. Next, unwind for ten to fifteen minutes, or until the mask dries.

Use your fingertips to rub the dried mask off your skin, simultaneously exfoliating it, and then wash off any remaining residue for a deeply cleaning facial. Rinse the mask off with warm water until the face is clean for a moisturizing facial.

How to Blend Them

The mask will only last for an hour or two, so only mix enough for one application. Any leftovers can be applied to the upper back, knees, or elbows. Combine all ingredients in a small dish and mix thoroughly with a teaspoon to make an essential oil mask. A powdered component is required to get the desired paste-like consistency. Top tiers include:

For A Moisturising Mask	For A Cleansing Mask
Ground Almonds	Bran
Rice Flour	Fuller's Earth
Oatmeal	Kaolin

If the oatmeal, bran, or almonds are too coarse, pulse them in a food processor to make them more finely ground before adding them to the mask. The finer the powdery ingredient, the more it will tighten and extract dirt from the skin. Any moisturizing mask will benefit from the addition of a teaspoon of melted, heated honey. Applying a heated washing mask beforehand will make it more visually appealing. Once the prepared paste is well warmed through, place it in a glass jar with a screw cover and place it in a container of just boiling water. The perfect concoction would be:

Cleansing	Moisturising
6 drops essential oil in 30ml (1fl oz/ 6 tsps) hot water mixed with enough powdery ingredient to make a smooth, thick paste	6 drops essential oil in 30ml (1fl oz/ 6 tsps) carrier oil mixed with enough powdery ingredient to make a sticky, thick paste

Masks For Trouble Spots

If you already have a face moisturizer and oil combination, you can easily prepare masks with it (see recipes in the chapter "ESSENTIAL OILS FOR THE Face"). Simply add enough of the powdered ingredient to create a paste. Alternatively, you can utilize one oil that is especially well-suited to skincare (see the list for the finest aromatic/therapeutic oils) and especially well-suited to your personal scent preferences.

Additionally, keep in mind that you can apply multiple masks in patches. For example, apply a moisturizing mask to dry cheeks, an oil-controlling mask to the nose and chin, and a firming mask to the jaw and neck. Applying a little amount of massage oil or a mixture of 15 drops rose oil to 30 ml (1fl oz/6 tsp) jojoba to the skin after the mask has been removed is an option. Before you start experimenting on your own, try these recipes for the most popular kinds of masks to ensure that you mix them perfectly.

Basic Face Masks

Moisturising mask

30ml (1fl oz/6 tsps) of apricot oil, 2 drops each of frankincense, rose, and neroli, 1 tsp of melted, warmed pure honey, and enough finely crushed almond to form a soft paste

Deep cleansing mask

In 30ml (1fl oz/6 tsp) hot water, combine 2 drops geranium, 3 drops lavender, and 1 drop lemon. Add enough kaolin to create a smooth paste.

Relaxing mask

30 ml (1fl oz/6 tsp) sweet almond oil, 2 drops each of violet, lavender, and neroli, and enough oats to form a smooth paste

Energising mask

30ml (1fl oz/6 tsp) of cooled water, 2 drops each of ylang-ylang, petitgrain, and lemon, and enough crushed almond to make a smooth paste

Anti-ageing mask

30ml (1fl oz/6 tsps) of evening primrose oil, 2 drops of neroli, mandarin, and orange each, 1 tsp of warmed, melted clear honey, and enough crushed almond to produce a smooth paste

Steam Facials

There's one more really efficient technique to use essential oils into your beauty regimen. Just include them into a steam face. This strategy offers two benefits. Essential oils are absorbed more quickly when steam opens pores and heats the skin. In addition, the oils become more volatile and evaporate more quickly, resulting in an even higher aromatic content than before. Additionally, the steam facial is speedy, mess-free, and incredibly soothing.

Some essential oils, meanwhile, are too strong to be directly inhaled in a confined space and absorbed with steam in this manner due to their potency, especially since they can irritate eyes and enter the nasal passages. Anyone with a history of respiratory issues, such as asthma, should avoid steam facials. The oils on the next page should not be used since they irritate the respiratory system when inhaled.

When to Use a Steam Facial

Steam facials can be used once a week at most to replace face masks for deep cleaning or deep moisturizing the skin. They instantly brighten skin, making them especially useful for dull, dry, oily, or spotty skin.

But avoid using them right before you have plans to leave the house because the heat and steam can leave your cheeks looking quite flushed and glossy for a few hours. It is preferable to use them right before bed because they are quite calming. Furthermore, whatever moisturizer you apply afterward will instantly become an even more effective night cream as it begins to operate on your softened, warmed skin.

Oils **NOT** Recommended For Steam Facials
Basil
Bay
Birch
Camphor
Citronella
Clary Sage
Fennel
Ginger
Juniper
Laurel
Pine
Tarragon
Tea-Tree
Thyme
Valerian

How To Use A steam Facial

Wear an off-the-shoulder top and make sure your skin is completely clean. Next, bring some water to a boil. Transfer the necessary quantity into a large dish that can hold heat and set it on a table. Ascertain that the height is appropriate for you to sit comfortably and lean forward over the bowl. To capture the steam, prepare a thick towel to drape over your head. Next, gradually add your preferred essential oils to the water's surface, drop by drop.Close your eyes and stay beneath the towel until the steam subsides. Then, pour extra hot water into the bowl to remove any last traces of essential oils. After that, massage your face dry gently and slather on a moisturizer right away to seal in the excess steaming water.

To make steam facials, mix one liter (2 pints) of boiling water with five drops of essential oil.

Steam Facials For Troubled Spots

When doing a steam facial, it's advisable to use no more than two distinct essential oils because the heat intensifies their aroma, making any more inevitably overbearing. However, practically any skin and psychological issue can be treated with the appropriate combination. Before you begin making your own mixtures, consider attempting these recipes:

Deep Cleansing Steam Facial

For dry skin

2 drops lavender and 3 drops of violet

For normal & mixed skin

2 drops mimosa and 3 drops geranium

For oily & blemished skin

3 drops juniper and 2 drops bergamot

For mature skin

3 drops frankincense and 2 drops galbanum

Deep Moisturising Steam Facial

For dry skin

2 drops chamomile and 3 drops of jasmine

For normal & mixed skin

2 drops rose and 3 drops sandalwood

For oily & blemished skin

2 drops chamomile and 3 drops geranium

For mature skin

2 drops of neroli and 3 drops rose

Relaxing Steam Facial

2 drops of ylang-ylang and 3 drops jasmine

Invigorating Steam Facial

2 drops of peppermint and 3 drops lavender

Chapter 6: Essential Oils for the Body

It is not appropriate to begin skin care from the neck up.
Actually, the skin on the rest of your body is identical to the skin
on your face; thus, because there is more of it, it requires more
care. Although most people acknowledge that their bodies aren't
ideal, they don't take many steps to make them
better.Nonetheless, compared to other beauty regimens, using
essential oils to the body produces greater results faster. This is
due to the fact that you can treat specific areas with readily
absorbed, low-cost, and highly effective made-to-measure
treatments.

Rather than purchasing a skin-smoothing exfoliant, you may
DIY it and incorporate an essential oil to simultaneously reduce
cellulite. Alternatively, you can make two types of moisturisers
using essential oils: one for treating your greasy back and
another for relieving dry skin on the rest of your body. This way,
you can avoid using an all-over body lotion.

Body Moisturisers

The greatest body treatment out there is definitely an essential-
oil moisturizing lotion. In order to get the most out of applying
essential oils, you should dilute them with a carrier oil. This will

help the oils spread evenly, dissipate gradually, and stay on the skin until they are absorbed. And what makes them such effective moisturizers is the carrier oil just as much as the fragrant ones.

All moisturizing creams function by preventing the natural water in your skin from evaporating into the atmosphere by sealing the skin's surface. The more oil in your moisturizer, the better, since oil, not water, is what provides the moisturizing benefit.

This is especially true for moisturizers for the body. The lack of sebaceous glands, which produce oil and keep skin naturally supple, is the reason why rough, dry patches frequently appear on the elbows, knees, and feet. But because there are so many sebaceous glands on the upper back, they frequently clog, resulting in spots and greasiness.

When To Use Them

When the proper therapeutic drops are added to pure oil for optimal moisturization, it's called an essential-oil body therapy. That's all there is to it. They are basic, pure, non-irritating, cheap, quick and simple to mix, and you can use them as often as you wish.

After a bath or shower, when skin is warm, damp, and somewhat swollen from the water, is the ideal moment to apply them. The skin then absorbs the essential oils more quickly. To test it, after taking a bath, rub a peeled clove of garlic into the sole of your foot and notice how soon you can detect the fragrance of garlic on your breath.Although most of us don't take two daily baths, it is recommended to apply body moisturizers in the morning and evening. The next best approach to accelerate the absorption of oil after it has been massaged onto the skin is to use body heat to warm the oil until it nearly melts into the skin. You can use the step-by-step invigorating body rub section in chapter "Essential Oils for Massage" to follow an entire routine that creates maximum heat and friction, or you can just rub the oils in with strong, rhythmic palm strokes.

How To Use Them

Since a broad region of warm skin needs to be moisturized with body oils, the oils should be diluted thoroughly. If not, the heat from your body may make them unbearably fragrant. To ensure that the carrier oil is completely absorbed, always apply them sparingly. If you smear yourself like a sardine, the oil will ruin your clothes and be squandered.Just enough should be combined to last a few days; the more fresh the components, the more advantageous they are. A teaspoon of wheatgerm oil or the

117

contents of a vitamin E capsule can be used as a natural preservative if you really must make a big batch. For body moisturizers, the recommended ratio is 15 drops of essential oil to 60ml (2fl oz/12 tsp) of carrier oil.

How To Blend Them

Selecting the appropriate carrier oil has a significant impact on the body moisturizer made of essential oils. Some are richer and more emollient, some are lighter and quickly absorbed, and some are especially beneficial for specific skin issues.

Pure, cold-pressed oils are always the finest option because they mix nicely with essential oils and are of the highest quality. Drop by drop, add the essential oils to a dark glass bottle after measuring out your preferred carrier oil. Before using, make sure to shake well and store in a cool, dark spot.

Best Carrier Oils For The Body	Use
Apricot Kernel	For Wrinkles
Evening Primrose	For Wrinkles
Olive Oil	For Rough Skin
Peanut	For Dry Skin
Safflower	For Oily Skin
Sesame	For Stretch Marks
Sunflower	For Oily Skin
Sweet Almond	For Normal, Itchy & Sensitive Skin

Best Carrier Oils For The Body	Use
Wheat Germ	For Scars

Making Your Own Body Moisturisers

You can choose to add scent for therapeutic purposes, enjoyment, or both when creating your own essential-oil body moisturizer. Use your nose to lead you if it's just for fun. Match your moisturiser to your bath oils if you use aromatherapy, as it's great to layer the fragrance. Applying little amounts of the therapeutic oils to specific difficulty areas is always an option. For the remainder of your body, apply an aromatic blend. Alternatively, if you combine the two, you'll look and feel better all at once.

Best Aromatic Oils For The Body
Geranium
Jasmine
Lavender
Mimosa
Neroli
Rose
Sandalwood
Violet

Best Therapeutic Oils For The Body	Benefits
Bergamot	For Oily Skin
Chamomile	For Itchy Skin
Cypress	For Cellulite
Frankincense	For Stretch Marks
Lavender	For Sensitive Skin
Myrrh	For Dry Skin
Rose	For Mature Skin
Tea-Tree	For Cracked & Rough Skin

Best Remedies For Moisturising The Body

To ensure that your concoctions will smell and function as beautifully as possible, refer to the charts for mixing oils and essential oil uses while creating your own recipes. Remember that the final scent needs to be pleasing to the nose because it will cover you from head to toe. Before you mix it together, if in doubt, use the blotting paper sniff test (see chapter "Introduction") to get a sense of the finished aroma. These are some great body moisturizing recipes to get you started in the right direction.

Rich Moisturisers

For mature skin

Remedy #1:

- 7 drops rose and 4 drops each lavender and sandalwood in 60ml (2fl oz/12 tsps) apricot kernel oil

Remedy #2:

- 4 drops galbanum, 5 drops geranium and 6 drops lavender in 60ml (2fl oz/12 tsps) sesame oil

For dry skin

Remedy #1:

- 8 drops myrrh and 7 drops rose in 60ml (2fl oz/12 tsps) peanut oil

Remedy #2:

- 5 drops each patchouli, sandalwood and jasmine i 60ml (2fl oz/12 tsps) sweet almond oil

For summer

Remedy #1:

- 4 drops each chamomile, lavender and sandalwood in 60ml (2fl oz/12 tsps) peanut oil

Remedy #2:

- 7 drops each rose and neroli in 60ml (2fl oz/12 tsps) grapeseed oil

For winter

Remedy #1:

- 5 drops each sandalwood, juniper and petitgrain in 60ml (2fl oz/12 tsps) olive oil

Remedy #2:

- 6 drops lavender, 4 drops frankincense and 4 drops myrrh in 60ml (2fl oz/12 tsps) of sweet almond oil

Light Moisturisers

For oily skin

Remedy #1:

- 8 drops lavender and 3 drops each lemon and petitgrain in 60 ml (2fl oz/12 tsps) sunflower oil

Remedy #2:

- 5 drops each bergamot, chamomile and geranium in 60ml (2fl oz/12 tsps) safflower oil

For itchy & sensitive skin

Remedy #1:

- 5 drops rose and 9 drops chamomile in 60ml (2fl oz/12 tsps) sweet almond oil

Remedy #2:

- 8 drops lavender, 2 drops marigold and 5 drops violet in 60ml (2fl oz/12 tsps) sweet almond oil

For summer

Remedy #1:

- 5 drops each bergamot, geranium and neroli in 60ml (2fl oz/ 12 tsps) safflower oil

Remedy #2:

- 6 drops rose, 4 drops jasmine and 5 drops mimosa in 60ml (2fl oz/12 tsps) sunflower oil

For winter

Remedy #1:

- 4 drops each sandalwood, patchouli and myrrh in 60ml (2fl oz/12 tsps) sweet almond oil

Remedy #2:

- 6 drops sandalwood and 4 drops each orange and ylang-ylang in 60ml (2fl oz/12 tsps) sunflower oil

Other Body Treatments

Numerous different treatment solutions can be made using the basic carrier-oil/essential-oil body moisturizing blend. Add some to a small amount of hot water for a great pre-manicure soak that softens nails. A grainy ingredient, such finely chopped almonds or coarse sea salt, can be added to create a smoothing and calming body exfoliant. Additionally, you can include fuller's earth, kaolin, or finely crushed oatmeal to thicken the mixture and use it as a body mask if you need to treat a particular area.

How To Blend Them

These treatments are great for treating problem areas on the body, and they're also quite affordable because you can mix exactly what you want and how much.

Body Exfoliator

For patches of very rough skin

Fill a screw-top glass jar with five heaping tablespoons of coarse sea salt. Pour in 5ml (0.2fl oz/1tsp) of body moisturizing lotion and stir, distributing the mixture over the salt in tiny drops. Shake the jar to combine, and let it sit overnight before using.

Rub into elbows, knees, and heels with slightly damp skin to remove tough, thick areas of skin. After using warm water to rinse, immediately apply a body moisturizer.

For dry or coarse skin

To form a smooth paste, finely chop or combine two teaspoons of fresh almonds and add enough body moisturizing mix. Two tablespoons of fresh almonds should be coarsely chopped and mixed into the paste. Apply right away.

Apply the paste to your buttocks, thighs, upper arms, upper back, shoulders, and any other dull areas of skin by rubbing it in circular motions while your skin is somewhat damp. Apply a thick body moisturizer to finish.

Body Pack

For a small area of skin

Place the glass bottle with the 10ml (0.4fl oz/2 tsps) body-moisturizer mix in a pot of boiling water. Next, incorporate with oatmeal until finely blended, creating a thick paste.

Perfect for dabbing dry areas of skin or splotchy areas of the back or chest. For a sketching effect, apply the paste while it's still heated and rinse it off once it cools.

For a large area of skin

Make a smooth, soft paste by combining 60ml (2fl oz/12 tsps) of body moisturizing mix with enough dried kaolin or fuller's earth. Apply right away.

Apply a small layer of the paste to the affected area and allow it to firm for cellulite, fluid retention, or varicose veins. After rinsing, rub a body moisturizer in.

Body Soak

For rough & hard skin

30ml (1fl oz/6 tsp) of the body-moisturizer mixture should be added to a small basin of hot water. Apply right away.

Apply prior to getting a manicure or pedicure. After soaking, apply a pumice stone right away to any extremely hard skin regions. Apply a body moisturizer to finish.

For thick & coarse skin

Pour 30ml (1fl oz/6 tsp) of the body-moisturizer mixture into a small amount of hot water. Apply it right away after soaking a cotton rag in it until it becomes sodden.

Great for easing stiff spots like knees, elbows, or other parts of the body before rubbing in a body moisturizer.

Top-To-Toe Trouble Spots

Because essential oils permeate the skin fast and effectively, they are great for treating any issues that are close to the skin. It is worth persevering by using the appropriate body oils morning and night for at least two weeks because all the common issue locations, from stretch marks to blackheads, respond extremely effectively. Here are some recipes for the most typical complaints about the appearance of the skin and body.

The Feet

For cold feet & poor circulation

3 drops each eucalyptus and ginger in 30ml (1fl oz/6 tsps) olive oil

For callouses & rough skin

3 drops each lavender and sandalwood in 30ml (1fl oz/6 tsps) olive oil

For athlete's foot, warts & corns

3 drops lemon and 4 drops tea-tree in 30ml (1fl oz/6 tsps) olive oil

The Knees

For thick & coarse skin

3 drops each rose and lavender in 30ml (1fl oz/6 tsps) olive oil

The Legs

For varicose veins

2 drops each cypress, lime and marigold in 30ml (1fl oz/6 tsps) sweet almond oil

For cellulite

4 drops each lavender, juniper and rosemary in 60ml (1fl oz/6 tsps) of sesame oil

For stretch marks

3 drops lavender and 2 drops each frankincense and sandalwood in 30ml (1fl oz/6 tsps) sesame oil

For fluid retention

3 drops cypress and 2 drops each geranium and sage in 30ml (1fl oz/6 tsps) sweet almond oil

The Arms

For slack skin on upper arms

2 drops each geranium, lemongrass and marjoram in 30ml (1fl oz/6 tsps) sesame oil

For dry skin on elbows

2 drops each chamomile, jasmine and sandalwood in 30ml (1fl oz/6 tsps) olive oil

The Hands

For nails

3 drops each bay and sandalwood in 30ml (1fl oz/6 tsps) sweet almond oil

For skin

2 drops each lavender, geranium and chamomile in 30ml (1fl oz/6 tsps) sweet almond oil

The Back

For spots & oiliness

2 drops each chamomile, bergamot and basil in 30ml (1fl oz/6 tsps) safflower oil

The Body

For scars

3 drops lavender and 2 drops neroli in 15ml (0.5fl oz/3 tsps) wheatgerm oil

For excessive perspiration

3 drops citronella and 2 drops each lemongrass and bergamot in 30ml (1fl oz/6 tsps) sunflower oil

For energy

2 drops each peppermint, rosemary and lemongrass in 60ml (2fl oz/12 tsps) sweet almond oil

For relaxation

7 drops each jasmine and neroli in 60ml (2fl oz/12 tsps) sweet almond oil

Chapter 7: Essential Oils in the Bath

The Romans spent hours socializing in hot springs, Cleopatra had baths in asses' milk, and Mary, Queen of Scots, favored taking a hot wine bath. Some of us take baths in salt water these days, while others utilize ice-cold water, jets, steam, sprays, spurts, or gurgles. Bathtime is the most peaceful moment of the day in a hectic world, regardless of the circumstances, thanks to the soothing combination of warm water, steam, and a soothing soak.

However, adding essential oils to your bath makes it a wonderful experience instead of just enjoyable. It is the most tranquil aromatherapy procedure available. The warm, steamy environment causes the oils to release more scent molecules than when you massage it, and the hot water helps to soften your skin and accelerate the absorption of the oils, making the effects of the essential oils more powerful for your body and mind.

If you utilize multiple essential oils, you'll find that the aroma is greater in warm, moist air, similar to the scent of a bouquet of flowers. Not only can you smell the entire bouquet with your eyes closed, but you can also identify each individual flower. Heat creates waves in the distinct oils, allowing you to smell each one alone and in combination. The end effect is an aroma so unique and exquisite that you will have a hard time identifying which oil is which.

The Essential Oil Bath

Before you undress, make sure everything is as cozy and pleasant as possible to get the most out of a fragrant bath. Additionally, keep in mind that you can achieve nearly any effect in the bath by using essential oils. They are especially beneficial for invigorating or soothing tense, dry, or sunburned skin; relieving muscle soreness, PMT, or cramps; and treating colds, hangovers, and headaches. Baths with flowers or citrus are especially refreshing in the summer. Green, spicy, or woody scents are the most comforting and calming in the winter.

The greatest all-arounders, available year-round, for adding a single oil to your bath are:

Best Oils For The Bath	Quantity	Benefits
Bergamot	5 Drops	For Melancholy, & Depression
Chamomile	7 Drops	For Insomnia & Itchy Skin
Frankincense	8 Drops	Sedative, Calming & Mood Sweetening

Best Oils For The Bath	Quantity	Benefits
Geranium	10 Drops	Relaxing but Uplifting & Energising
Jasmine	8 Drops	For Apathy, Stress & Fatigue
Lavender	10 Drops	Relaxing, Soothing & Positive
Neroli	8 Drops	Hypnotic & Anti-Depressant
Patchouli	5 Drops	Energising & Invigorating
Rose	10 Drops	Romantic, Brings Happiness & Pleasure
Sandalwood	8 Drops	Intimate, Sensual & Mellowing

Basics Of Bath Time

To retain as much aroma in the space as possible when applying essential oils, make sure the bathroom door is closed and the faucets are off. Drop by drop, add essential oils to the water until they float there. As you walk into the tub, the oils will mingle and cover your skin.

Refrain from adding too much oil, even if you will only be able to smell the aroma for a short while. The scent of the oils will continue to evaporate for at least fifteen minutes, but the human nose quickly grows used to it and ceases to detect it.

Additionally, it's common for lesser doses of essential oils to have a bigger effect than larger ones, so don't assume that using twice as much will relieve your headache twice as quickly. It won't, and using oils in excessive concentrations runs the danger of causing skin irritation.

Key Elements Check-List:

- Lots of big, cozy towels

- Gentle, atmospheric lighting

- A wrapped towel or a neck cushion

- Calming eye pads

- Phone switched off

- Room at warm and cozy temperature

How Many Drops

A bath should generally contain a maximum of ten drops of essential oil, although some of the stronger-smelling oils, like rosemary, eucalyptus, peppermint, bay, basil, lime, and lemon, can get by with just five drops. Use one oil alone or combine up to three different oils for your bath; however, don't use more than this since the advantages will just cancel each other out.

Choosing Oils

Select oils that have complementary or comparable benefits. They can be classified into three basic categories: therapeutic, soothing, or exciting (according to the chart provided). You can add therapeutic oils to either of the other two types, but combining stimulating and calming oils together could negate their beneficial effects separately.

Refer back to the oil mixing at-a-glance chart and the directory of common problems (see chapter "Essential Oils for Common Problems") if you need assistance selecting which particular oils to use. This list of tried-and-true bathtime remedies will encourage you to try more on your own and will help you relax your body, mind, and spirit all at once.

Relaxing Baths

In summer & hot weather

Remedy #1:

- 4 drops lavender, 4 drops neroli and 2 drops geranium

Remedy #2:

- 4 drops mandarin, 4 drops geranium and 2 drops pine

In winter & cold weather

Remedy #1:

- 3 drops sandalwood, 3 drops ylang-ylang and 2 drops pine

Remedy #2:

- 4 drops patchouli, 2 drops ginger and 2 drops frankincense

To conclude a hard day

Remedy #1:

- 5 drops rose and 5 drops lavender

Remedy #2:

- 3 drops chamomile, 3 drops geranium and 2 drops patchouli

For her

Remedy #1:

- 3 drops rose, 3 drops jasmine and 4 drops neroli

Remedy #2:

- 3 drops ylang-ylang, 3 drops sandalwood and 3 drops jasmine

For him

Remedy #1:

- 3 drops pine, 2 drops chamomile and 2 drops lemon

Remedy #2:

- 4 drops frankincense, 2 drops basil or 3 drops sandalwood

Invigorating Baths

In summer & hot weather

Remedy #1:

- 2 drops each basil, patchouli and juniper

Remedy #2:

- 3 drops rosemary, 3 drops mint and 3 drops lemon

In winter & cold weather

Remedy #1:

- 3 drops eucalyptus, 3 drops clary sage and 2 drops mint

Remedy #2:

- 3 drops petitgrain, 3 drops bergamot and 2 drops lemon

To conclude a hard day

Remedy #1:

- 5 drops patchouli and 4 drops mint

Remedy #2:

- 4 drops rosemary, 4 drops thyme and 2 drops mint

For her

Remedy #1:

- 4 drops ylang-ylang and 4 drops petitgrain

Remedy #2:

- 2 drops each mint, clary sage and basil

For him

Remedy #1:

- 3 drops rosemary, 3 drops mint and 2 drops juniper

Remedy #2:

- 4 drops each thyme and basil

Therapeutic Baths

Bath for coughs & colds

Remedy #1:

- 3 drops pine, 2 drops lemon and 2 drops tea-tree

Remedy #2:

- 3 drops eucalyptus, 3 drops lavender and 2 drops mint

Bath for dry & itchy skin

Remedy #1:

- 5 drops lavender and 5 drops chamomile

138

Remedy #2:

- 4 drops rose, 4 drops chamomile and 2 drops jasmine

Bath for aches & pains

Remedy #1:

- 4 drops eucalyptus, 3 drops clary sage and 3 drops thyme

Remedy #2:

- 3 drops marjoram, 2 drops ginger and 4 drops rosemary

Bath for insomnia

Remedy #1:

- 2 drops each ylang-ylang, rose, lavender and neroli

Remedy #2:

- 3 drops chamomile, 2 drops camphor, 2 drops juniper

Bath for headache & hangover

Remedy #1:

- 5 drops each rose and lavender (plus some ice folded in a towel to use as a neck pillow)

Remedy #2:

- 2 drops mint, 2 drops lemon and 4 drops marjoram

Aquatherapy

You can change the style of bath simply by adjusting the water temperature: tepid or warm water for a pleasant, long, skin-wrinkling soak; very hot or very cold for an in-and-out speedy bath. You can also obtain a therapeutic benefit from the essential oils you use. Aromatherapy can be used after aquatherapy. An aromatherapy massage or body moisturizing treatment thereafter will be even more beneficial if you take a simple bath devoid of essential oils to soften skin, warm muscles, and relax them.

Warm water is calming, tepid water makes you sleepy, hot water makes you weak and floppy, and cold water stimulates. Thus, after nightfall, after a demanding day, is the ideal time for a soothing bath. To get you going in the morning, an energizing one is a fantastic choice. When you arrive home exhausted and need to unwind but still have the energy to go out again, you can utilize aquatherapy to blend the two water temperatures.

Starting with a warm or hot bath is the most gentle approach to mix hot and cold water without experiencing goosebumps. After a thorough soak, empty the bath, turn on the cold water faucet, and allow the water to slowly refill. You may feel the hot and cold water whirling about your body independently when the cold water is running by swirling the bathwater with your hand.

You won't be shivering after the bath is finished; instead, you'll feel revitalized and eager to depart.

Temperature tips:

- A cool bath (65-75°F/18-24°C) is the most invigorating & energising pick-me-up

- A tepid bath (75-85°F/24-30°C) is the most soporific & gentle

- . A warm bath (85-95°F/30-35°C) is the most deeply relaxing & soothes aches

- A hot bath (95°F/35°C or more) is slightly debilitating & leaves you weak. Avoid them when you are pregnant, if you have varicose veins, if you suffer heart problems or high blood pressure

Best Oils For A Cold Bath	Best Oils For A Hot Bath
10 Drops Geranium	6 Drops Chamomile
5 Drops Lemon	8 Drops Frankincense
8 Drops Mimosa	10 Drops Lavender
5 Drops Pepper Mint	8 Drops Neroli
8 Drops Violet	6 Drops Ylang-Ylang

The Essential Oil Shower

It's not quite as relaxing to use essential oils in the shower as it is in the bathtub. A large amount of the oil and its scent escape through the plughole because the water is constantly running. Aromatic showers are the most effective approach to stimulate your body and mind because it is quite hard to unwind completely when standing up!

Mixing essential oils with a carrier oil beforehand and massaging them in before you step under the spray is the easiest method to prevent wasting them in the shower. Alternatively, you can use a sponge dipped in the mixture to massage your body as you take a shower. Your shower will smell better if it has a deep base since the oils will vaporize in the warm water at the bottom of the shower when the plug is blocked.

Best Oils For The Shower
Basil
Bergamot
Lemongrass
Lime
Mandarin
Orange
Peppermint

The Footbath Or Mini Bath

More strain is placed on the feet than practically any other area of the body. They may dance all night and then have to bear all that weight during the day. Giving them a relaxing foot bath is the best treat you can give them. It promotes blood circulation, eases aches and pains, releases blocked nerves, and warms and relaxes all of the little support muscles.

It can be made even more enjoyable with the correct essential oil. In addition, you get to breathe in the scent molecules and take in a quiet moment throughout a hectic day because you have to sit while you soak. A sizable bowl or square pail, warm water, a towel that is warm, a seat that is at the most suitable height for relaxation, and the appropriate essential oils are all you need. Simply add them to the water drop by drop before dipping your feet in. For every nine liters (two gallons) of water, you can use up to eight drops.

Footbaths and handbaths come in particularly handy if you are too old or disabled to take a complete bath with essential oils, or if you just can't take a full bath at all.

Stimulating Footbaths

Remedy #1:

- 2 drops bay and 4 drops of ginger

Remedy #2:

- 4 drops citronella and 4 drops angelica

Relaxing Footbaths

Remedy #1:

- 5 drops basil

Remedy #2:

- 3 drops lavender and 3 drops geranium

Therapeutic Footbaths

For aching feet

Remedy #1:

- 4 drops thyme and 4 drops chamomile

Remedy #2:

- 4 drops eucalyptus and 3 drops pine

For athlete's foot

Remedy #1:

- 3 drops birch and 6 drops geranium

Remedy #2:

- 8 drops tea-tree

Excessive sweating

Remedy #1:

- 6 drops lemongrass

Remedy #2:

- 4 drops bergamot and 4 drops citronella

146

Chapter 8: Essential Oils for Common Problems

Based on their overall properties, essential oils fall into three basic categories. There are oils having a medicinal impact, oils that are stimulating, and oils that are soothing and relaxing.

A detailed chart that provides a brief overview of which herbs fit into each of the three categories can be found at the end of the book. The chart will direct you to essential oils like ambrette seed, juniper, laurel, and lavender if you're looking for one that will relieve your backache while also having a calming impact.

It is easiest to go straight to the appropriate entry in the alphabetical table of frequent problems included in this chapter if you are looking for a therapy for a specific condition. This provides you with additional details about particular illnesses or problems that you can cure using essential oils.

For example, you may read the entry under the letter "B" further down if you'd like more information about treating burns. You will learn about the nature of burns and how to treat them with essential oils from this. Each entry includes a list of the best oils for treating that condition. This highlights the general effects of each oil (whether it is relaxing, stimulating or healing), and points out any special features of the oils. In the entry on burns, you will discover that burns can be treated with lavender and tea-tree oils, both of which can be applied undiluted. For specific information on diluting, combining and mixing the different essential oils, turn to the chapter "How to Use Essential Oils". Before beginning your treatment, make sure to review these rules. It's critical to use essential oils correctly because some can be hazardous if used improperly.

ABRASIONS, CUTS & NAPPY RASH

Essential oils are incredibly effective at relieving minor cuts and skin abrasions, ranging from shaving nicks to diaper rash, by soothing and disinfecting the area.

Best Oils: chamomile, bergamot, lavender, citronella, tea-tree (anti-bacterial, antiseptic & anti-viral); geranium, marigold (soothing & healing).

ACNE (see also SKIN)

The excessive production of oil in the sebaceous glands is the cause of acne and skin outbreaks. Hormonal variations (typically caused by puberty, menstruation, or the menopause), poor food, inactivity, stress, worry, and anxiety all exacerbate the illness. Sebum surplus accumulates in hair follicles and greasy regions near the nose and chin. Because essential oils are not only antiseptic, antibacterial, and therapeutic, but they also relieve mental tension, which exacerbates acne, they are very useful for treating problem skin.

Best Oils: bergamot, cedarwood, geranium, juniper, lavender, lemon, rosewood, sandalwood, yarrow, tea- tree (antiseptic, healing & oil regulators); chamomile and petitgrain (for boils & inflammation); patchouli, lemongrass (cleansing).

ANXIETY (see also STRESS)

The stresses and strains, demands, disturbances, and worries of daily life are the root causes of anxiety. The symptoms can include sadness, low resistance, sleeplessness, headaches, and stiff, knotted muscles. Essential oils are beneficial because they lessen bad emotions, calm the body and mind, and elevate mood.

Best Oils: ambrette seed, mimosa, lavender, mandarin, neroli, patchouli, sandalwood, spruce, valerian (calming); bergamot, frankincense, rosewood, violet (uplifting & cheering); jasmine, petitgrain, clary sage, ylang-ylang (relaxing but uplifting).

ARTHRITIS

Inflammation of the joints is known as arthritis. There are two types: osteo-arthritis, which is caused by the wearing away of cartilage and causes pain, swelling, and loss of mobility, and rheumatoid arthritis, which affects the surrounding connective tissue and causes pain, swelling, and stiffness. Essential oils can alleviate pain, lessen inflammation, and relax muscles, but they cannot treat either illness.

Best oils: marjoram, ginger, eucalyptus, juniper, peppermint, pine (warming & relaxing); cypress, lime, myrrh, spruce, ambrette seed, lemon, rosemary (anti- inflammatory & healing).

ATHLETE'S FOOT & FUNGAL INFECTIONS

A fungal infection of the feet is known as athlete's foot. The skin in between the toes peels, gets red, and irritating. It is extremely contagious and is frequently contracted from the damp floors of public restrooms and showers, where the fungus grows.

Best oils: lavender (antiseptic & healing); tea-tree (anti-fungal), geranium, birch (anti-inflammatory & soothing); lemongrass (deodorising & drying).

BACKACHE

Almost everyone has experienced muscle and back discomfort at some point in their lives. It could be brought on by sneezing forcefully, lifting large weights, poor posture, exercising too much or too little, falling, or even pregnancy.

Best Oils: bay, camphor, citronella, eucalyptus, marjoram, pine, spruce (relaxing & warming); ambrette, petitgrain, juniper, rosemary (soothing & stimulating); lavender, clary sage, thyme (relaxes muscles & anti- inflammatory).

BITES AND STINGS

Essential oils are effective against insect bites and stings. The ones that are antiseptic and anti-inflammatory aid in lowering inflammation, swelling, and itching.

Best Oils: chamomile, lavender, marigold, peppermint, tea-tree, basil, citronella (soothing, anti- inflammatory & antiseptic).

BREATHING PROBLEMS & RESPIRATORY INFECTIONS

Frequent symptoms of respiratory disorders such as bronchitis, influenza, and sinusitis include copious mucus production, persistent coughing, constricted chest, and labored breathing.

Essential oils can ease breathing and coughing, open up the chest, and lessen congestion.

Caution: Use essential oils only after seeing your physician if you have a history of severe respiratory issues or asthma.

Best Oils: angelica, myrrh (coughs); cedarwood, marjoram, sandalwood (soothing & calming); eucalyptus, peppermint (decongestant); pine, tea-tree, rosemary (anti-viral).

BRUISES

A bruise indicates tissue damage, typically from a bump or knock. Long after the initial agony subsides, a discoloration that is purple, black, or yellow is caused by blood seeping from injured capillaries.

Best Oils: camphor and clary sage (warming & increases circulation); geranium, calendula, marjoram (soothing); lavender, cypress (anti-inflammatory).

BUNIONS

A bunion is an excruciating swelling of the joint between the big toe and the foot that is typically brought on by wearing shoes that are too small.

Best Oils:

peppermint (refreshing & soothing); cypress (anti-inflammatory); lemon (circulation boosting).

BURNS AND BLISTERS

Skin that comes into contact with something hot gets burned. Blisters and inflammation that ensue are more prone to infection. Essential oils' antimicrobial, antiviral, and antiseptic qualities aid in promoting natural healing while shielding the affected area during the growth of new skin.

Best Oils: lavender, tea-tree (soothing, healing & antiseptic, both can be applied undiluted to burnt skin immediately); chamomile, geranium, marigold, rose (soothing & healing).

CELLULITE

The scourge of many women's existence, cellulite is a lumpy, dimpled, orange-peel-textured skin condition that affects the thighs, bottom, and backs of arms. It is believed to be brought on by an accumulation of toxins and fluid in the tissues as a result of irregular hormone levels and impaired circulation. Frequent application of essential oils to the skin might help reduce the lumpy texture.

Best Oils: juniper, geranium (detoxifying); rosemary, fennel (diuretic); bay, cypress, lemon, lime, spruce, cedarwood (circulation boosting); lavender, sage, patchouli (decongestant).

CHICKEN POX

The childhood sickness that is so painful that it is best not to scratch the affected areas. Essential oils are quite helpful since they lessen itching and prevent the pox virus from spreading.

Best Oils: tea-tree, eucalyptus, bergamot, lavender (soothing, antiseptic & healing); chamomile (soothing & anti-itch).

CHILBLAINS

After being exposed to extremely cold temperatures, swollen, discolored veins develop on the fingers, toes, and backs of legs, which are known as chilblains.

Best Oils: ginger, spruce, eucalyptus (warming & soothing); cypress, marjoram, rosemary, juniper, tea- tree, lemongrass, lemon (circulation boosting).

CIRCULATION, POOR

The main causes of poor blood circulation are sedentary lifestyles, prolonged periods of inactivity, and lack of exercise.

Essential oils can assist to improve blood flow, lessen cellulite, warm hands or feet that are too cold, and give the skin a more radiant, healthy look.

Best Oils: basil, cedarwood, cypress, spruce, ginger, juniper, lemon, lemongrass, lavender, myrrh, pine, peppermint, rosemary, clary sage, bay, ambrette seed, ylang-ylang (stimulate circulation); lime, marigold (varicose veins).

COLDS

In the winter, the common cold is nearly unavoidable due to its high contagiousness. A high temperature, pains, sore eyes, sore throat, coughing, sneezing, and congestion in the chest and nose are some of the symptoms, which are brought on by a variety of constantly evolving viruses. While there is currently no recognized scientific cure for the cold, essential oils can aid with some of these symptoms.

Best Oils: peppermint, eucalyptus, lavender, lime, pine, tea-tree, lemon, marjoram (decongestant, & anti- viral); angelica, thyme, camphor, bay, myrrh, spruce (relieve sinus congestion), laurel (strengthens resistance).

COUGHS & RESPIRATORY INFECTIONS

Anybody can become distracted by an unpleasant cough, which can be brought on by anything from dust to cigarette smoke to allergies to the typical cold. Essential oils inhaled work wonders to relieve a cough. Actually, the primary ingredient in a lot of prepared drugs like Vicks Vaporub and Karvol is aromatherapy oil.

Best Oils: angelica, atlas cedarwood, eucalyptus, peppermint, myrrh, thyme, sandalwood, spruce (expectorant & anti-viral); frankincense (calming & relaxing); ginger, rosemary (decongestant); pine, cedar, cypress, lemon (anti-viral).

CRAMPS

The worst times of the night to get cramps are frequently when the menstrual cycle is starting, poor circulation, excessive exertion, or a vitamin deficit. Essential oils relieve pain, ease tight muscles, and, if necessary, help you fall back asleep.

Best Oils: eucalyptus, lemon, marjoram, mandarin (warming, relaxing); juniper (boosts circulation); jasmine, laurel, tarragon, fennel (for period cramps); ambrette seed, rose, lavender, ylang-ylang, neroli, chamomile (relaxing & soporific).

DANDRUFF

Dandruff is a result of an imbalance in the oils at the surface of the skin, which is brought on by hyperactive sebaceous glands. It manifests as either sticky, oily scales or tiny, dry flakes on the scalp. Both kinds are scratchy, bothersome, and frequently get infected. Dandruff is a great condition to treat, and essential oils can generally get rid of all the symptoms.

Best Oils: tea-tree (anti-inflammatory, oil regulating & antiseptic); bay, birch, juniper, cedarwood, lemon and rosemary (antiseptic & astringent); lavender, geranium, sandalwood (soothing & antiseptic).

DEPRESSION

Because life is full of ups and downs, most people discover that their happy times are counterbalanced by depressive ones. While feeling depressed is common, it can also cause insomnia, fatigue, and general misery. Because smell is recognized in the same area of the brain as memories, moods, and emotions, essential oils are very effective at modifying your mood.

Best Oils: clary sage, sandalwood, geranium, lavender, ylang-ylang (relaxing & uplifting); jasmine, rosewood, neroli, rose, mimosa, bergamot (energising & uplifting); frankincense (for confidence); myrrh (dispels dark moods).

DERMATITIS, ECZEMA & PSORIASIS

Every year, allergic skin inflammations occur more frequently. Given that contemporary life exacerbates stress, anxiety, exhaustion, and pollution, perhaps this rise is the result of modern living. Many of the symptoms, especially inflammation, itching, and infection, can be reduced with the use of essential oils, which are great skin healers and soothers.

Best Oils: birch, bergamot, cedarwood, chamomile, cypress, violet lavender, geranium, myrrh (healing); marigold (soothing & anti-inflammatory); (contact dermatitis & psoriasis); sandalwood (extra-dry skin).

FATIGUE

More people than anything else lament their lack of sleep. It's probably a combination of too much work, too many obligations and stressors, and not enough downtime or leisure. Essential oils are highly beneficial because they can induce a state of mental and physical relaxation that prepares you for enjoyment rather than sleep.

Best Oils: ambrette seed, eucalyptus, lemongrass, rosemary, peppermint, thyme, ginger, lemon (stimulating); basil, bergamot, clary sage, galbanum, jasmine, lavender (de-stressing

& uplifting); fennel, orange, patchouli, geranium, frankincense (gently relaxing).

FLU

Compared to the average cold, influenza is a more dangerous viral infection that sends most individuals home for a few days. Certain symptoms of the flu can be relieved and the virus from gaining too much hold on the body by using essential oils.

Best Oils: eucalyptus, lime, rosemary, peppermint (clear head congestion); pine, tea-tree (anti-viral); thyme, spruce, marjoram (expectorant & decongestant); laurel, orange (boost the immune system).

FLUID RETENTION

It appears that men experience fluid retention only after extended airplane travel. Most women experience it when they are pregnant, having their period, or just from being on their feet all day. Applying the appropriate essential oils to the area will help to minimize swelling.

Note: As stated in the chapter "How To Use Essential Oils", certain essential oils should not be used while pregnant. First, speak with your physician.

Best Oils: birch, juniper, rosemary, fennel (diuretic); cypress (relieves pre-menstrual swelling); mandarin, patchouli, geranium, spruce (stimulating & boost circulation).

HAIR LOSS & ALOPECIA

A few months following childbirth or illness, severe stress, abrupt shock, or using certain drugs can all cause temporary hair loss. Baldness, or permanent hair loss, is typically inherited. While essential oils can aid in hair thinning, they are sadly powerless to cover a bare scalp.

Best Oils: rosemary, bay, ylang-ylang (rejuvenating & circulation stimulators); lavender, cedarwood (tonic & stimulating) sage, yarrow (promotes hair growth).

HAIR, greasy

Excessively active sebaceous glands in the hair follicles are the source of greasy hair, which looks lank and lies flat to the head. Stress, menstruation, pregnancy, menopause, and adolescence all cause hormonal changes that exacerbate the issue. By controlling oil production without being overly astringent or drying out the scalp, an essential oil scalp massage (see the detailed procedure in the chapter "Using Essential Oils For Massage") might be beneficial.

Best Oils: tea-tree, lemon, lavender, geranium (astringent & oil regulators); rosemary, bay, cypress (cleansing & tonic).

HAIR, dry & split

A weekly essential oil scalp massage will help moisturize and smooth out dry hair (see the detailed method in the chapter "Using Essential Oils For Massage"). Avocado or olive oil make the greatest carrier oils. Apply after warming 30ml (1fl oz/6 tsp) of carrier oil and adding 5 drops of the selected essential oil. Before shampooing out, let it sit overnight.

Best Oils: chamomile (for blonde hair); rosemary, lavender (red & brown hair); bay (dark hair); tea-tree, bergamot (dandruff).

HANGOVER

After consuming too much alcohol the previous morning, take an aromatherapy bath to relieve your headache, nausea, and fatigue. Use an ice pack as a neck pillow as you recline, and sip lots of water.

Best Oils: geranium, rose, lavender, neroli (soothing & uplifting); peppermint, lemon (clears the head, energises & reduces nausea).

HEADACHE & MIGRAINE

A headache could indicate that the head is at its breaking point. If you lie in a darkened area and inhale essential oils, they can help reduce tension, anxiety, lights, and activity. For more information, check the chapter "Inhaling Essential Oils." Alternatively, if it's tolerable, try giving yourself a little scalp massage (refer to the detailed instructions in the chapter "Using Essential Oils For Massage").

Best Oils: eucalyptus, peppermint, lemongrass (clear the head); lavender, violet, ambrette, rose, chamomile (relaxing & analgesic), frankincense, clary sage, thyme (relieve tension).

HERPES & COLD SORES

The herpes virus is responsible for shingles, genital herpes, cold sores, and blisters that hurt and reoccur frequently. Certain essential oils, however, can calm them and hasten the healing process.

Best Oils: tea-tree, marigold, bergamot, lavender, lemon (healing & anti-viral); chamomile (soothing); eucalyptus and patchouli (antiseptic).

HOUSEHOLD CLEANING

Essential oils are used in a lot of modern chemical disinfectants and household cleaners. These oils are selected for their antibacterial, antifungal, and fresh scents in addition to their antiseptic qualities. Consider a dishwashing liquid with lemon flavor or a pine scent. Two of the most popular aromatherapy oils for fighting germs are pine and lemon. See the chapter "Inhaling Essential Oils" for ideas on how to use the best essential oils for disinfection around the house.

Best Oils: lavender, geranium, tea-tree, chamomile, bergamot, citronella, lemon, lime, lemongrass, thyme, eucalyptus, peppermint, pine.

INDIGESTION

Heartburn, gas, and indigestion are typically caused by eating too rapidly and in excess, having a spicy or rich diet, or going for extended periods of time without eating at all. Relief can be achieved by massaging gentle, clockwise circular strokes into the stomach with essential oils. Or use a tissue to inhale the scents.

Best Oils: angelica, fennel, lavender, peppermint, marjoram, tarragon (aches & digestives); ambrette, mandarin (warming & relaxing).

INSECT REPELLENTS (see also BITES AND STINGS)

During the summer, insects can take over the entire house. They will come out of cracks and crevices, jump across carpets, fly through windows, and land on any warm flesh or clothing. Essential oils fear anything little with more than two legs and make wonderful natural, aromatic, non-toxic pesticides. Refer to the chapter "Inhaling Essential Oils" for information on using them at home.

Best Oils: camphor, lemongrass (moths & most other insects); citronella (mosquitoes); basil, tea-tree, thyme (ants, fleas & most flying insects).

INSOMNIA (see also STRESS)

It's quite annoying, draining, and upsetting to be unable to fall asleep, but worrying and counting sheep while you lie there won't make it better. Enjoy a relaxing aromatherapy bath during this time. You'll discover that the best oils are those that have sedative or peaceful properties.

Best Oils: basil, chamomile, cypress, geranium, lavender, mandarin, neroli, rose, mimosa, petitgrain, marjoram, valerian, jasmine, sandalwood, ylang- ylang, yarrow (calming & sedative).

JETLAG

It's interesting to think about the days when flying was a glamorous endeavor. Now, when most people think of air travel, they picture jet lag—that disorienting feeling that occurs at the beginning of your vacation when you can't sleep at your destination, can't get off the plane, have swollen feet, dehydrated skin, lack of appetite, can't finish sentences, can't find your luggage, etc. Essential oils come to the rescue. Use geranium oil to help you go asleep and lavender oil to help you stay awake when you land to help you acclimate to time differences more quickly.

Best Oils: lavender (reviving); geranium (relaxing & calming); cypress (for swelling); peppermint (head clearing).

MEASLES

Even the sweetest youngster can become an unhappy little moaner due to the measles's uncomfortable, itchy rash and foul mood. Furthermore, the symptoms of measles in adults are 100 times more severe. Apply the appropriate essential oil to the skin and massage it in gently.

Best Oils: bergamot, lavender, eucalyptus, tea-tree (soothing, antiseptic & uplifting); chamomile (anti-itch & relaxing).

MENOPAUSE

The natural decline in oestrogen and progesterone hormones, which marks the end of the reproductive years, initiates the menopause. It can start at any point between the ages of 40 and 60, and while many women experience minimal changes, others deal with a wide range of uncomfortable symptoms, such as profound melancholy and stomach discomfort, hot flashes, and low self-esteem.

Best Oils: chamomile, rose (rebalancing); lavender, cypress, geranium (regulate hormone production); peppermint, clary sage, ylang-ylang (anti-depressant),

NAUSEA

Being ill is the only thing worse than feeling ill. Rich or spicy foods, tainted food, a bad odor, stress, anxiety, traveling in motion, pregnancy, or migraines are common triggers. A small amount of essential oil inhaled through a tissue is very beneficial.

Note: Before using aromatherapy to relieve nausea during pregnancy, refer to the list of essential oils that should be avoided in the chapter "How To Use Essential Oils" and speak with your doctor.

Best Oils: peppermint, lemon, ginger, mandarin (settle the stomach).

PRE-MENSTRUAL TENSION (see also CRAMPS)

A collection of symptoms known as pre-menstrual tension can be brought on by hormonal fluctuations anywhere from two days to two weeks before to the menstrual cycle. Some women experience severe problems with headaches, nausea, edema, breast and abdominal fluid retention, illogical behavior, moodiness, and depression. When used in a bath or massage, essential oils can improve mood and relieve a variety of physical ailments.

Best Oils: geranium, lavender, rose, chamomile, sandalwood (calming, balancing & uplifting); bergamot, jasmine, juniper, clary sage (emotionally hormones); cypress, fennel, tarragon, laurel (fluid retention & cramps); peppermint (energising).

RHEUMATISM

Rheumatism typically affects the knees, ankles, hips, and wrists and produces discomfort in the surrounding muscles, ligaments, and soft connective tissue. Warming the muscles, reducing inflammation, and relaxing tissue are all assisted by essential oils.

Best Oils: angelica, birch, rosemary, juniper, cypress, lavender, eucalyptus, lemon (anti-inflammatory); chamomile (analgesic); angelica, thyme, ginger, lime, pine spruce, marjoram (warming & relaxing).

SEXUAL PROBLEMS

You know your life has reached a tipping point where fatigue and stress have replaced passion with exhaustion when you find yourself diving into bed to sleep instead of play. Essential oils are excellent in relieving tension and allowing you to feel euphoric or drowsy.

Best Oils: ylang-ylang, clary sage, ginger, jasmine, neroli, patchouli (relaxing & sensual aphrodisiacs); rose, rosewood (romantic & aphrodisiac); sandalwood, geranium (relaxing & uplifting).

SKIN

Essential oils are ideal for daily skincare routines since they are affordable, quickly absorbed, thoroughly penetrate the skin, easy to apply, fragrant, and pleasant. They also work wonders for treating a wide range of skin conditions.

Mature Skin

The natural renewal process of young skin takes about thirty days, but as we age, this process slows down and our skin loses its delicate, youthful bloom. Premature wrinkling and skin aging can be exacerbated by stress, smoking, pollution, alcohol, too much sun exposure, and insufficient physical activity. Essential oils are great moisturizers and help prolong the suppleness and smoothness of skin.

Best Oils: rose, neroli, orange, geranium, lavender, frankincense, ylang-ylang, rosemary (skin rejuvenators); chamomile, galbanum (soothing & healing).

Thread Veins

Tiny red lines called thread veins can be seen on the cheek and leg skin. Poor circulation, exposure to the sun or wind, and heavy alcohol use are the causes.

Best Oils: rose, chamomile, geranium (anti- inflammatory & soothing); marigold, cypress, violet, lemon, lime, orange, yarrow (vascular constrictors & calming).

Dry & Sensitive Skin

Alcohol, central heating, excessive sun or wind exposure, underactive sebaceous glands, and poor skincare practices can all contribute to dry skin. Essential oils that are calming and moisturizing can both protect and hydrate skin.

Best Oils: rose, sandalwood, neroli, marigold, geranium (moisturising); jasmine, lavender, chamomile, violet (sensitive skin); myrrh, tea-tree, patchouli (cracked & rough skin).

Greasy & Blemished Skin

The overproduction of sebaceous glands in greasy skin leads to spots, blackheads, and open pores from the extra oil. The soothing and somewhat astringent essential oils work wonders and can even control the skin's natural oil production.

Best Oils: chamomile (soothing & cleansing); lemon, lime, bergamot, mandarin, cedarwood, juniper, geranium (rebalancing & antiseptic); neroli, lavender (healing); lemongrass, petitgrain (open pores); violet, patchouli, thyme (blackheads).

STRESS

Our complex, contemporary lifestyle includes stress, which is brought on by undue demands on our time and energy. It can cause severe sickness and manifest as allergies, sleeplessness, anxiety, sadness, tenseness, and irritability in addition to muscle aches and pains. Essential oils that are energizing, calming, and relaxing are quite helpful.

Best Oils: jasmine, basil, neroli, rosewood, geranium, bergamot, sandalwood, ylang-ylang, rose, frankincense, galbanum (anti-stress & uplifting); marjoram, mandarin, clary sage, valerian, lavender, chamomile, patchouli (calming & sedative).

SUNBURN

These days, we should avoid becoming sunburned because it ages skin and increases the risk of cancer. If you do burn, though, essential oils can help speed up your skin's natural healing process while also relieving and cooling the burn itself.

Best Oils: lavender, chamomile, geranium, rose (soothing & anti-inflammatory).

SWEATINESS & PERSPIRATION

The regulating, deodorizing, cooling, and antibacterial properties of essential oils might help manage excessive sweating or sweatiness. See the chapter "Essential Oils For The Body" for suggestions on how to use the oils.

Best Oils: bergamot, citronella (reduce excessive perspiration); lemongrass, lavender, thyme (anti- bacterial & deodorising).

THRUSH, CANDIDA & FUNGAL PROBLEMS

Tea tree oil is the most effective essential oil for treating vaginal or genital fungal infections because of its extraordinary, recently discovered antiviral, antifungal, and disinfecting qualities. It doesn't irritate delicate vaginal tissue and is safe to use. Use a solution of one part essential oil to ten parts warm water to douche or bathe the afflicted area. Other antiseptic oils have the ability to heal, calm, and lessen itching.

Best Oils: tea-tree (anti-fungal); juniper, lavender, myrrh, sandalwood (antiseptic).

TRAVEL SICKNESS

Transport sickness is typically brought on by motion sickness from flying, sailing, or land transport, but it can also be brought on by a genuine fear of traveling.

Best Oils: peppermint, ginger, lemon, mandarin (calming & settle the stomach); bergamot (uplifting & soothing).

Chapter 9: The A-Z Directory of Essential Oils

This Directory has been put together to provide you with all the knowledge you could possible require regarding essential oils, their characteristics, and the advantages they provide. It also directs you toward the oils that you will enjoy the most on a personal level. It indicates which oils blend well together, eliminating the need for guesswork when combining oils. Additionally, it outlines the specific oils that are most effective for various health or lifestyle issues.

How to Utilize This Listing

It can be used from any point of reference that you have. The alphabetical list of the 48 most popular essential oils in this chapter will show you what lavender oil does. It includes information about each oil's origins, herbal traditions, qualities, aromatherapy actions, common uses, and any necessary safety precautions.

The chapter "Essential Oils For Common Problems" contains an alphabetical list of issues, from abrasions to travel sickness, along with a list of the essential oils that will assist fix them. If you have a headache and can't be bothered reading through all

48 essential oils to find out which works best, turn to this chapter.

See the at-a-glance specific chart at the end of the book for a summary of the best uses for each oil type and how useful they are overall.

Utilize the chart that illustrates which oils mix well together if you are unsure whether the small recipe you are creating with essential oils will smell sweet or merely sickly sweet (see the specific chart at the end of the book).

Ambrette Seed (Abelmoschus Moschatus)

The fully ripened, musky, kidney-shaped seeds are used to extract oil. The evergreen shrub is grown in China, Indonesia, and the West Indies, where it thrives.

In the East, ambergris seed is pulverized and consumed as a spice. It is also used in fragrance as a musk alternative. It has historically been used to treat headaches, nerves, and stomach problems like cramps, indigestion, acidity, and other stomach issues.

The essential oil smells rich and musky and has calming and energizing qualities. It is said to be aphrodisiac and is soothing and warming.Aromatherapy works well for disorders like

174

anxiety, depression, exhaustion, and other stress-related issues. Additionally, it helps with poor circulation, cramps, and muscle aches.

Use: compress, inhale, massage, and take a bath. A few drops on a tissue will help reduce headaches and nausea from travel or morning sickness, as well as clear your head whether you're feeling under the weather or just mentally exhausted. Foot fatigue can be relieved with four drops in a basin. Use sparingly in the bath or for massages.

Caution: If diluted before application, ambrosia seed oil is completely safe for usage at home.

Angelica (Angelica Archangelica)

The plant's seed, fruit, or root are used to extract oil. It is native to Europe and is grown in Belgium, Hungary, and Germany.

The most well-known usage of angelica is in cake decorating as the green, candied stem. During the plagues of the 14th and 15th centuries, the root was traditionally eaten and burned to prevent infection and treat coughs and indigestion.

The smell of the essential oil is musky, spicy, and earthy. It is an excellent digestive and good expectorant, and it relieves rheumatic diseases, gas, and colic.

175

It is a powerful germ-killer in aromatherapy and works wonders for colds, coughs, the flu, rheumatism, and muscle aches. It is warming and relaxing, and it calms the digestive system.

Use: compress, inhale, massage, and take a bath. A few drops on a tissue will unclog your nose, and inhaling steam will ease the congestion of a smoker's or chesty cough. Indigestion can be relieved, sore joints and muscles can be soothed, and cuts and bruises can heal more quickly when five drops are added to the bath or mixed with two tablespoons of carrier oil and massaged in.

Caution: Because the root oil is phototoxic, it is best to protect your skin from the sun after using it to prevent irritation. Not to be taken when expecting.

Basil (Ocimum Basilicum)

Sweet basil that is in flower is used to extract oil. It is now grown commercially throughout America, the Mediterranean, the Pacific Islands, and Europe.

For generations, basil has been regarded as an aphrodisiac and is a staple in most diets. It is still worn tucked in the hat to frighten away insects in Mediterranean climes, where it was originally believed to fend off evil spirits.

The essential oil smells warm, fragrant, sweet, and spicy, with a very high camphor content. It's a bright, cheery, and refreshing tonic. Aromatherapy treats bug bites, headaches, poor circulation, aches and sprains in the muscles, nervous sleeplessness, anxiety, and fatigue.

In bug bites, headaches, poor circulation, aches or sprains in the muscles, nervous sleeplessness, anxiety, and fatigue, aromatherapy treats them all.

Use: Inhalation, baths, and massage. The head is cleared with a few drops on a tissue. When diluted with massage oil, it can be applied topically to ease aches and pains or insect bites. Additionally, taking a bath scented with fragrant basil will cheer you up.

Caution: Always use basil with caution as it can be strong and cause skin sensitivity in certain individuals. Steer clear of when pregnant.

Bay, West Indian (Pimenta Racemosa)

The dried leaves and berries of the bay rum tree are used to extract the essential oil. Originally from South America, it is currently farmed in the West Indies, including Barbados and Jamaica.

In the past, hair tonic was traditionally made by steeping West Indian bay leaves in rum. This moderately antiseptic remedy, once believed by the Victorians to cure hair loss, is now acknowledged to aid with oily hair and flaky scalps.

The essential oil smells warm and invigorating, with a manly, woodsy, clove-like aroma. It has astringent and antibacterial qualities.

It works wonders as a scalp stimulant in aromatherapy, drawing blood to the surface of the skin and eliminating oil from hair. It is also beneficial for cellulite, aches in the muscles, and poor circulation.

Use: As a poultice, massage, inhalation, and compress. It works best when used sparingly in conjunction with a friction massage to enhance the circulation-boosting effects, especially on the scalp, over tense, stiff shoulders, on sore muscles or cellulite areas, and to warm hands or feet that have been chilled by the cold. When steam is used, it can be inhaled to treat infections of the nose, throat, or chest.

Caution: Because bay might irritate the mucous membrane, use it sparingly. Eugenol, its primary ingredient, can corrode metal, thus it's best to store it in a dark, glass bottle.

Bergamot (Citrus Aurantium Bergamia)

The bitter orange fruit that is almost ripe is peeled to obtain oil. Nowadays, Sicily, Morocco, southern Italy, and other parts of Africa grow it for economic purposes.

Southern Europe has been using bergamot since the 16th century as a fever remedy. The flavor of Earl Grey tea comes from bergamot, which is also frequently used as a scent and fixative in toiletries, cosmetics, and sun care products.

The essential oil has antibacterial, invigorating, and revitalizing properties. It smells clean, somewhat spicy, and has a hint of warm balsamic.

Depression, melancholy, exhaustion, irritability, stress, acne, and oily skin are all treated with aromatherapy. It works well as a deodorant and will help eradicate germs from the house.

Use: Inhalation, massage, and baths. A room can be made to smell better by placing a few drops in a saucer of hot water on top of a radiator. It also has antibacterial qualities and a lovely smell. It can be immediately breathed from a tissue to treat emotional distress or depressive states. Use a small amount (up to five drops) for a massage or to brighten your mood when taking a bath.

Caution: Skin may become irritated by bergamot oil, particularly if it is later exposed to sunlight. If properly diluted, it can be used safely at home.

Birch - White (Betula Alba)

The white birch tree's bark and leaf buds are used to extract oil. It is grown in Finland, Sweden, Germany, and northern Russia.

For generations, birch has been used as a remedy for rheumatism, arthritis, and skin issues. In order to produce a fragrant steam that will deep clean the skin and increase circulation, Scandinavians hang little bundles of the leafy branches in their saunas.

The essential oil has diuretic, antibacterial, anti-inflammatory, and calming properties. It smells warm, leathery, and woodsy.

It works wonders for fungal infections, eczema, dandruff, and dry skin in aromatherapy. It also aids in reducing fluid retention and cellulite.

Use: Baths and massages. Massage into the stomach, thighs, and buttocks after diluting with a carrier oil to help break down stubborn cellulite or lessen the "bloat" associated with pre-menstrual tension. Apply a few drops to a warm bath or massage it into particularly dry areas of your skin. Additionally, a few drops added to a heated footbath will relieve fungal diseases like athlete's foot.

Caution: If diluted before application, birch essential oil is completely safe for usage at home.

Camphor - White (Cinnamomum Camphora)

The evergreen camphor tree's wood, stumpy roots, and tender branches are all used to produce oil. Although it originated in China, Taiwan, and Japan, it is currently grown as far away as California and India.

Traditionally, people have worn camphor around their necks to protect against contagious illnesses, bad luck, and to fortify their hearts. It has been used for a very long time as a pesticide, especially in moth balls.

The heated, strong smells emanating from the essential oil are caused by the presence of terpenic ketone. For sprains or aches and pains in the muscles, it works well.

It works well in aromatherapy to relax tense, sore muscles, ease mild sprains, and ease stiff necks. Also, it keeps most insects away.

Use: Massage. Applying camphor topically to sore or hurting muscles should be done cautiously and with great dilution. A cotton ball or the hem of curtains or blinds treated with a few drops works wonders as an insect repellent, especially for flies and moths.

Caution: Asthmatics should avoid breathing in the strong odors of camphor oil. If properly diluted and given to targeted areas only, as opposed to the entire body, it can be safely used for massage.

Cedarwood - Atlas (Cedrus Atlantica)

The wood of the evergreen coniferous tree is used to extract oil. The best essential oil nowadays originates in Morocco, however it was originally from Lebanon.

Because cedars are believed to bring longevity, they are typically planted in cemeteries. The oil that the trees produce was used as incense in Tibet and the East, and embalming in ancient Egypt. It is supposed to treat skin conditions like eczema and baldness.

The scent of the essential oil is woodsy, like shavings from a lead pencil. It has an astringent, tonic impact and is invigorating and refreshing.

Dandruff, thinning hair, dermatitis, rashes, eczema, oily skin, and acne can all benefit from aromatherapy. It also aids in the symptoms of any stress.

Use: Baths and massages. Apply a small amount of oil or a few drops to a basic moisturizing lotion and massage into dry skin. To give yourself a steam facial for oily skin, add a few drops to a basin of boiling water and bend over it while covering your head with a towel. It's also a great oil for massaging the scalp.

Caution: If Moroccan cedarwood is diluted before application, it is completely safe for usage at home. Pregnancy is the greatest time to avoid it, though.

Chamomile - German (Matricaria Recutita)

The newly dried, daisy-like blossoms are used to extract oil. The plant is cultivated throughout North America and Eastern Europe.

One of the earliest herbs used for medicine and cosmetics in Britain is chamomile. It was once said to 'cure all agues'. The most effective uses of it were to lighten blonde hair, as a great disinfectant in World War II, and as a tea to soothe sleeplessness.

Rich in azulene, a naturally occurring anti-inflammatory and restorative ingredient, is the essential oil. It smells like straw and apples and has calming sedative properties.

Stress, insomnia, headaches, rashes, bug bites, burns, cuts, toothaches, and menstruation or menopausal issues are among the conditions for which aromatherapy is utilized.

Use: compress, inhale, massage, and take a bath. Put ten drops of oil in a warm bath to help you unwind after a stressful day. It can be applied topically and applied as a compress for menstruation discomfort or headaches after being diluted with a carrier oil. It works wonders as a home disinfectant as well.

Caution: If diluted before usage, chamomile essential oil is completely safe for use at home.

Citronella (Cymbopogon Nardus)

Freshly dried tropical grass is used to extract oil. The best types are from Sri Lanka, Java, and the Seychelles, where it grows naturally near the sea.

Traditionally, citronella leaves were applied topically to treat fever, discomfort, and to hasten the healing process. It is well known as an outstanding insect repellent throughout East and Southeast Asia, and it was used in China to treat rheumatic pain.

The essential oil smells even more strongly like lemon and has excellent antibacterial properties. It has a strong deodorizing effect and is beneficial for aches and pains.

It works well in aromatherapy for rheumatic issues, sprains, and soreness in the muscles. It improves mental alertness and works wonders as a germicide and antibacterial.

Use: compress, inhale, and take baths. You can burn the oil in a room to destroy germs and freshen the air, or you can use a few drops on a tissue to clear your brain. It relieves aches and works wonders to stop excessive sweating when applied as a poultice. Applying a small amount of diluted oil directly to mosquito or other bites helps reduce itching and serve as an antibacterial. A few drops on your bedding may also deter insects.

Caution: As long as citronella is well diluted before application, it is completely safe for use at home. Pregnancy is the greatest time to avoid it, though.

Cypress (Cupressus Sempervirens)

The evergreen tree's cones, twigs, and freshly harvested leaves are used to extract oil. Although it originated in the Mediterranean, it is now grown all throughout Europe and North America.

The ancient Greeks held the cypress tree in high regard. The Egyptians utilized it for medical purposes and to create sarcophagi. It is now recognized to be an effective vascoconstrictor and has a history of relieving internal hemorrhage.

The essential oil smells warm, woodsy, and balsamic and has an energizing, refreshing impact. It increases circulation, is antiseptic, and is astringent.

It works wonders in aromatherapy for issues related to menstruation or menopause, varicose or damaged veins, fluid retention, cellulite, and to ease a chronic cough.

Use: compress, poultice, inhalation, massage, and baths. When diluted with a carrier oil, it can be used as a leg warming hand or foot massage, a fantastic abdomen-to-thigh massage for fluid retention, and an excellent massage for varicose veins. A few drops on a pillow will halt coughing, and it works well as a poultice for menstruation aches or swelling.

Caution: Dilute cypress before applying it to ensure complete safety for home use.

Eucalyptus (Eucalyptus Globulus)

The Blue Gum tree's twigs and leaves are used to extract oil. Originally from Australia, it is currently grown in California, Portugal, and Spain.

The Aborigines crushed eucalyptus leaves and used them to treat wounds, prevent infections, and ease pain in their muscles. To flavor meals, the wood was utilized in cooking fires.

The essential oil has been used for decades in cough and cold medicines because of its unique, energizing scent that clears the head. It is an effective antiseptic that cools skin and eliminates airborne bacteria.

It works wonders as an aromatherapy decongestant for fever, the flu, coughs, colds, and sinuses. It helps abrasions heal and relieves aches, strains, and pains in the muscles.

Use: Poultice, inhalation, massage, and baths. Apply a few drops to a hot water dish on a radiator to freshen the air and facilitate breathing at night. You can also use it as a hot compress, in a steamy bath, or as a massage oil for your chest. It can be used diluted to sore spots on the body to provide prompt relief.

Caution: Dilute eucalyptus before applying it to ensure complete safety for household use.

Fennel (Foeniculum Vulgare)

The crushed seeds of the sweet fennel plant are used to extract oil. It is grown in portions of India, Germany, France, and Italy.

The Egyptians, Chinese, Indians, and Greeks utilized fennel to provide longevity, strength, courage, and power. It is traditionally used to treat eye infections, stomach issues, and to help nursing moms produce more milk.

The essential oil smells sweet and peppery like anise and works well as an antibacterial, diuretic, tonic, and digestive. It's a typical component in baby gripe water.

When used in aromatherapy, it works well for stomachaches, cramps, fluid retention, PMT, and fatigue, especially the kind that results from overdoing physical activity.

Use: compress, poultice, inhalation, massage, and baths. A warm bath with a few drops will invigorate you. Alternatively, put some straight into a tissue and take a whiff for a quick pick-me-up. For any stomach issues or digestive concerns, dilute it and massage it in, or apply it with a warm compress.

Caution: If sweet fennel is carefully diluted and used sparingly, it is quite safe to use at home. Those who have epilepsy or are pregnant shouldn't use it.

Frankincense (Boswellia Carteri)

Oil is derived from the tree's gum resin. Originally from the Middle East and Africa, the resin is now gathered as far afield as China before being processed in Europe.

Frankincense has been valued for generations and was one of the three gifts given to the baby Jesus in addition to being burned as the first incense to please the gods. Numerous cultures employed it to cure nearly every known illness.

The aroma of the essential oil is rich and warm, with a hint of lemon and woodsy camphor. It has energizing, soothing, and moderately antibacterial properties.

Aromatherapy works wonders for fatigue, irritability, low moods, insecurity, and emotional upheaval. It provides a relaxing effect and aids in slowing breathing.

Use: Inhalation, massage, and baths. A few drops used to massage oil will warm, soothe, and revitalize a body that has been overworked or overstressed. Tension headaches can be relieved by massaging the scalp and temples. To relieve tension and elevate your mood, either inhale it straight or incorporate it into a soothing bath.

Caution: As long as frankincense is diluted before application, it is completely safe to use at home.

Galbanum (Feurla Galbaniflua)

The enormous fennel plant's gum resin is used to extract oil. In North Africa and southern Europe, it is farmed economically.

For centuries, galbanum has been utilized. The Hebrews used it as an anointing oil, and the Egyptians used it for embalming. It was also a component of early cosmetics and incense. It has historically been healing, soothing, and used to cure skin and stomach issues.

The scent of the essential oil is slightly melon-like, woodsy, and warm. It is invigorating, quiet, peaceful, and incredibly revitalizing.

It works well in aromatherapy for mending skin that is blemished, scraped, or scarred. Additionally for nervous tension, weariness, stress, tension, or anxiety.

Use: Inhalation, massage, and baths. When combined with additional aromatic essential oils, it creates a deeply calming and revitalizing body massage or bath, as well as a therapeutic facial massage for skin imperfections. Although it is not the most pleasant smell when inhaled alone, it has a tonic effect.

Caution: As long as galbanum is well diluted before application, it is completely safe to use at home.

Geranium (Pelargonium Graveclens)

The perennial shrub's fresh blooms, stalks, and leaves are used to extract oil. Madagascar, Egypt, Spain, France, Italy, Russia, and the Congo are among the countries where it is grown.

One of the most popular garden plants nowadays, geraniums blossom in a riot of colors and spread their tangy, sweet scent throughout the world. Although geranium oil was found in the 1850s, its near sibling, robert, has long been utilized in herbal medicine.

The smell of the essential oil is rosy-sweet with notes of lemon and mint, and it offers calming and tonic properties for the nervous system. It soothes skin well and has a slight antibacterial effect.

It's one of the most essential oils in aromatherapy; it can help you feel happy, sleepy, energized, or completely relaxed. Cuts, bruises, eczema, burns, acne, broken veins, and dry or older skin can all benefit from it.

Use: compress, inhale, massage, and take a bath. To hasten healing, apply a single drop immediately to lacerations or bruises. It is incredibly calming when added to a hot bath and invigorating when added to a cold one. It works great for a headache, neck and shoulder, or facial massage when combined with a carrier oil.

Using geranium at home is completely safe.

Ginger (Zingiber Officinalis)

The dried root of the tropical herbaceous perennial is used to extract oil. It is grown in Florida, Africa, India, Japan, and the West Indies.

Ancient Greeks, Romans, Indians, Chinese, and Japanese people all employed ginger in their cuisine and medicine. It was especially advised for digestive problems and upset stomachs, although its warming properties also aid in lowering fevers.

The essential oil smells like lemon, pepper, and woodspice and has antibacterial, stimulating, warming, and astringent qualities.

Aromatherapy is beneficial for increasing circulation, relieving tense, chesty coughs, stomachaches, stiffness, or weariness. It works well to warm and revitalize weary feet because of its astringent and antibacterial properties.

Use: Poultice, inhalation, massage, and baths. Apply it topically on sore muscles, stomachaches, and coughs. Inhale it through a tissue to help cleanse the head and energize the body. The warming effect makes it especially useful for massage and baths in chilly weather.

caution: Ginger is very strong, so use it sparingly for baths and massages and never apply it directly to skin.

Jasmine (Jasminum Officinale)

The reason jasmine oil is so expensive is that it takes approximately eight million hand-picked flowers to extract one kilogram of oil before daybreak. It is grown in India, Italy, France, Egypt, and Morocco.

Above all, jasmine has long been valued for its sensual, exotic, and rich aroma that uplifts the spirits of anybody who inhales it. Due to its sensuous tone, it has long been utilized in toiletries and may be found in most great, classic perfumes.

The bright red color of the essential oil and its pleasant scent make it valuable in perfumery. It is energizing, soothing, and will impart confidence, optimism, and a hint of euphoria in you. It works well for any aches or cramps as well as dry or sensitive skin.

Aromatherapy works wonders for sadness, anxiety, exhaustion, agitation, and indifference. It is a great skin softener and beneficial for pre-menstrual tension as well.

Use: compress, poultice, inhalation, massage, and baths. Jasmine is a great addition to any soothing bath or massage because it blends nicely with most other oils. To make everyone feel calm, add a few drops to a saucer of water and set it on a radiator.

Caution: If jasmine essential oil is diluted before application, it is completely safe to use at home.

Juniper (Juniperus Communis)

The fresh berries and needles of the evergreen Juniper tree are used to extract oil. It is cultivated commercially in Scandinavia, Italy, France, Spain, and Canada. It is native to northern Europe.

Ancient Greeks and Egyptians utilized juniper berries to protect against illnesses, while in England, juniper was burned to frighten away witches and devils. These days, gin is most frequently flavored with the berries.

The essential oil has a piney scent with a hint of heat and pepper. In addition to being invigorating but calming, diuretic, and antibacterial, it works wonders for aches and pains.

Cellulite, cramps, fluid retention, menstruation issues, and sluggish circulation respond well to aromatherapy. Additionally, it has a relaxing impact on people who are too stressed and a toning effect on greasy skin or acne.

Use: compress, poultice, inhalation, massage, and baths. It is the perfect massage oil when diluted with a carrier oil for rheumatism, sore joints or muscles, and pre-menstrual tension or menstrual issues. A few drops added to the bath can provide a calming and uplifting soak. A sickroom is an ideal place to burn it as a germ killer.

Caution: Juniper can cause labor, thus it should never be used while pregnant. However, if diluted properly, it is absolutely safe to use at home.

Laurel (Lauarus Nobilis)

The evergreen tree's leaves are used to extract oil. It is grown in France, Italy, Greece, and the Balkan nations.

The laurel tree was thought to be gods' protection by the ancient Greeks. In their mythology, the young Daphne fled from Apollo by changing into a laurel tree. The Romans appreciated it as well; following his military triumphs, Caesar wore a laurel crown. It has been utilized as a culinary herb and potent remedy since ancient times.

The essential oil smells strongly of medicine with a hint of warmth and spice. It has antibacterial, warming, calming, and immune-stimulating properties.

Aromatherapy can help with pains, aches, cramps, and fluid retention. Building up your resistance is beneficial if you are prone to recurring colds, the flu, or other viral diseases.

Use: As a poultice, massage, or inhalation. To assist combat viral infections, place some oil in a dish of hot water on a bedroom radiator and bend over a basin of hot water to breathe in the steam. Use as a massage oil to ease aches, chest issues, fluid retention, and premenstrual tension.

Caution: Due to its potential to irritate delicate skin, laurel should only be used sparingly and highly diluted. Should not be utilized during pregnancy.

Lavender (Lavandula Augustifolia)

The evergreen shrub's flowering tips are used to extract oil. It is grown in southern Europe, as well as in Australia and the United Kingdom.

Ancient Romans loved lavender as a bathtime cleaner and employed it to expedite healing. It has been a component of soap, fragrances, talc, and potpourri since the 18th century.

Among the most widely utilized is the essential oil. Calming, refreshing, invigorating, and elevating the spirits, it is a potent antibacterial and healer that is simultaneously energizing and calming.

Aromatherapy works wonders for aches and pains, skin issues, tension, fatigue, and depression. It is safe to use during pregnancy and, because of its delicate nature, can be administered undiluted to burnt skin or bug bites.

Use: compress, poultice, inhalation, massage, and baths. A few drops in a hot bath will reduce anxiety and leave you feeling wonderfully sleepy. It will revitalize and rejuvenate you in a chilly bath. To help you feel better and clear your head, inhale a few drops from a tissue. It helps with stiff muscles and mental exhaustion during massage.

Using lavender essential oil at home is completely safe.

Lemon (Citrus Limon)

The citrus tree's fresh fruit rind is used to extract oil.
Commercial cultivation takes place in California, Florida,
Portugal, Spain, Italy, and Israel.

The British Navy employed lemons to prevent scurvy and the
ancient Romans used them to soothe upset stomachs and
sweeten their breath. Today, lemons are used for virtually
anything, from colds and sore throats to a slice of ice in a glass
of fizzy water.

The essential oil is stimulating, energizing, astringent,
deodorizing, diuretic, and antibacterial. It smells fresh and
tangy like citrus.

Whether you have a cold or are psychologically tired,
aromatherapy can help cleanse your thoughts, energize your
body, improve circulation, treat cellulite, or warm your hands
and feet.

Use: Poultice, inhalation, massage, and baths. On a chilly night,
a few drops in a warm bath will improve circulation. Breathe it
in through a tissue to combat fatigue or ease cold symptoms.

Apply it to a rag and use it to freshen up the smell in the sickroom or throughout the house.

Caution: Lemon essential oil can irritate skin, especially if it is exposed to sunlight just after application. Use it sparingly. Keep the container cold and dark.

Lemongrass (Cymbopogon Citratus)

Wild grass, either fresh or dried, is used to extract oil. Commercial cultivation of it takes place in Africa, the West Indies, India, and Sri Lanka.

Since lemongrass has been used to treat fever in India for ages, it is also known as fevergrass. In addition, it has long been burned to eradicate germs and used to treat skin conditions. These days, its primary use is in food, drink, and toiletry flavoring.

The essential oil is deodorizing, antiseptic, antibacterial, calming, therapeutic, and has a pleasant, lemony, grassy scent.

It works well in aromatherapy for open pores, boils, athlete's foot, headaches, excessive sweating, poor circulation, and insect repellent.

Uses: It will improve the compress for massage, baths, inhalation, poultice, irritated skin, armpits, feet, and hands. When thoroughly diluted and used topically to irritated areas such as the hands, feet, and armpits, it promotes circulation, accelerates healing, and eliminates odors. Apply the oil directly to shoes or trash cans to deodorize them, and on curtain hems to keep insects away. A few drops in a footbath or handbasin will help to warm the extremities and lessen perspiration.

Caution: As long as lemongrass essential oil is properly diluted, it is completely safe to use at home.

Lime (Citrus Aurantifolia)

The unripe citrus fruit's peel (Citrus Aurantifolia) is used to extract oil. Lime trees are now farmed in Florida, Mexico, Italy, and the West Indies for their oil.

Limey got his moniker from the fact that, like lemons, limes were historically provided to British sailors who ate the fruit to lower their chance of contracting scurvy. These days, it is a flavoring for food and beverages and a fragrance for cleansers and male grooming products.

The essential oil smells strongly of sweet citrus peel and is a good tonic and warming stimulant in addition to being antiseptic, antiviral, and antibacterial.

Aromatherapy is beneficial for conditions including oily skin, varicose veins, rheumatism, arthritis, poor circulation, cellulite, colds, flu, fever, or infections.

Use: as a poultice, massage, bath, or inhalation. It works well as an astringent face, diluted and applied to the chest for colds, or as a leg, anti-cellulite, or warming friction massage. It's a great way to take a refreshing, revitalizing bath in the summer or a great way to warm up in the winter. It can be breathed for any respiratory issues or congestion, or applied as a poultice for fever.

Caution: Use lime essential oil sparingly as it can irritate skin, particularly if skin is exposed to sunlight shortly after application. Keep the container cold and dark.

Mandarin (Citrus Reticulata)

The peel of the ripe citrus tree fruit is used to extract oil. Although it originated in southern China and the Far East, it is currently cultivated for oil in Florida, the West Indies, Brazil, Mexico, and Italy.

The fruit, which did not arrive in Europe until the 1880s, was traditionally given as a gift to the Mandarin lords of China for generations, hence the name Mandarin. These days, it flavor food and beverages and adds scent to cosmetics like perfume.

The essential oil smells delicious like oranges and lemons and has soothing, sedative, and digestive properties.

Aromatherapy uses it to treat scars, stretch marks, fluid retention, stress, restlessness, sleeplessness, and nervous tension.

Use: Inhalation, massage, and baths. It reduces stretch marks and makes a superb slimming massage for the thighs, hips, and buttocks. When you're feeling stressed or exhausted, inhale a few drops off a tissue or add a few drops to a hot bath for a profoundly calming and energizing soak.

Caution: Use mandarin essential oil sparingly as it can cause skin irritation, particularly if skin is exposed to sunlight shortly after application. Keep the container cold and dark.

Marigold (Calendula Officinalis)

The herb is used to produce oil from its blossoms. It is a native of the Mediterranean and is farmed commercially in northern Europe, Morocco, France, Bulgaria, and Hungary.

Calendula, sometimes known as marigold, has been used for ages as a folk treatment to strengthen weak eyes, soothe the heart, and lift the spirits. These days, it is applied on dry, cracked, or sensitive skin, varicose veins, and diaper rash.

The essential oil is a calming, very therapeutic substance with a musky, woodsy, and slightly disagreeable fragrance.

It works best in aromatherapy to cure and soothe cuts, burns, eczema, itching, and excessively dry, irritated, or sensitive skin. Additionally, it works well for sunburns, rashes, and insect bites.

Use: Baths and massages. Marigold is a wonderful healer, although it is best used sparingly because of its overpowering odor. For skin issues, add a few drops to a warm bath or dilute with a carrier oil and massage in.

Caution: If sufficiently diluted prior to application, calendula essential oil is completely safe for use at home.

Marjoram (Origanum Majorana)

The dried blooming heads of the plant are used to extract oil. Originally from Asia, it is currently planted throughout Europe, with oil crops being grown in Tunisia, Morocco, Germany, Hungary, and Egypt.

Greece saw marjoram as a representation of unwavering love, and India and Egypt considered it to be sacred. It was employed by all ancient civilizations to treat respiratory, neurological, and digestive ailments.

The essential oil is calming, soothing, warming, and nourishing. It smells spicy, peppery, like camphor and thyme.

Aromatherapy can help with lumbago, bronchitis, coughs, colds, bruises, aches, pains, sprains, tension, headaches, and insomnia.

Use: Inhalation, massage, and baths. A few drops in a warm bath improve mood, increase circulation, and relieve aches and pains in the muscles. When it comes to massage, it works especially well for sore necks, headaches, migraines, painful joints, muscle pain, and soreness from heavy exercise. To ease congestion or a chesty cough, inhale it while steaming.

Caution: If marjoram is well diluted before application, it is completely safe to use at home. It should not be used when pregnant.

Mimosa (Acacia Dealbata)

The tree's vibrant, pom-pom-like blossoms and twig ends are used to extract oil. Although it originated in Australia, it is currently grown in France and Italy in Europe.

For millennia, Australian Aborigines have used the 'wattle' tree for medicinal purposes, especially to cure injuries, infections, diarrhea, and upset stomachs. These days, the tannin-rich bark is employed by the leather industry.

The essential oil smells sweet, honey-like, green and flowery, and it possesses astringent, antibacterial, calming, and relaxing properties.

Aromatherapy uses it to treat despair, melancholy, emotional disturbance, over-sensitivity, and any type of nervous tension. It is also very helpful for general skin care.

Make use of baths, massages, and inhalations. When used with a warm bath, it creates a rejuvenating soak that will calm your mind and body simultaneously. It makes a nice massage for the face, neck, and scalp. Additionally, adding a few drops to a bowl of hot water on a radiator will make the people inside feel happy.

Caution: As long as the essential oil is well diluted before usage, mimosa essential oil is completely safe for use at home.

Myrrh (Commiphora Myrrha)

Resin that is taken from the tree's stem and shoots is used to make oil. It grows in the Middle East, northern India, and North Africa.

One of the three gifts that were given to the baby Jesus was myrrh, which was highly valued in ancient perfume, religious rituals, and medicine. It was applied topically to wounds, chest issues, embalming, and incense.

The aroma of the essential oil is rich, spicy, and camphorous. It has anti-inflammatory, antibacterial, astringent, warming, soothing, and healing properties. It is also a good expectorant.

In aromatherapy, it works wonders for treating eczema, old skin, arthritis, poor circulation, and any congestion in the chest or nose.

Use: Inhalation, massage, and baths. Myrrh's rich scent and warming properties make it an ideal choice for a wintery oil. In a bath, a few drops reduce stress. Alternatively, massage it over your face to prevent wrinkles, your hands to relax, your feet to warm, or any dry skin. It is a good expectorant and soothes a chesty cough when inhaled via a tissue or while steaming.

Caution: Myrrh essential oil is completely safe to use at home as long as it is thoroughly diluted before usage. It is not, however, advised to be used when pregnant.

Neroli (Citrus Aurantium Bigaradia)

Freshly harvested bitter orange tree blooms are used to extract oil. Sicily, North Africa, France, and Italy are the commercial growing regions for it. It was believed that Neroli oil was called after Anne-Marie, Princess of Neroli, who lived in Italy, and it was discovered in the late 1600s. When the Roman god Jupiter married Juno, he gave her an orange, and ever since, brides have carried the flower to ease anxiety.

The essential oil smells just like a beautiful, bitter-orangey blossom in the wild. It is an antidepressant, hypnotic sedative, and calmant.

In aromatherapy, it works wonders for relieving tension and stress of any kind, as well as for aging or dry skin, anxiety, insomnia, and anxieties.

Use: Inhalation, massage, and baths. Neroli is a natural tranquilizer, so combine it with other calming oils to create the most delightful bath you've ever imagined. In addition to being great for soothing massages of the back, scalp, neck, face, hands, and feet, it also enhances the texture of the skin. It is a perfectly safe oil to use when expecting. And to feel joyous even in the midst of hardship, sniff a few drops on a tissue or fill your home with the soothing, alluring aroma.

Using neroli essential oil at home is completely safe. Citrus oils should be kept in a dark, cool place to ensure their freshness.

Orange (Citrus Sinensis)

The fresh fruit peel of the sweet orange tree is used to extract oil. Although the tree is found all over the world, the major producing regions for oil are Brazil, Florida, California, Israel, France, and Italy.

Chinese medicine makes considerable use of oranges. To lessen hangovers, the Romans drank orange-flower water after orgies. It has been used to prevent colds and strengthen the immune system.

Because over 90% of the essential oil is limonene, it stimulates and refreshes while still leaving you feeling calm. As a skin rejuvenator, it is. excellent

When used in aromatherapy, it works wonders for soothing restless or exhausted people, including children. Apply it on wrinkles, sun-exposed skin, or a lifeless, pallid complexion.

Use: compress, poultice, inhalation, massage, and baths. It can be used for any facial massage or for massages when you need to unwind after a demanding day but still have the energy to go out that evening. It works wonders as a body moisturizer and soothes agitated kids when added to the bath.

Caution: Use orange essential oil sparingly because it can irritate skin, especially if skin is exposed to the sun shortly after application. Keep the container cold and dark.

Patchouli (Pogostemon Cablin)

The bushy herb's dried leaves and shoots are used to extract oil. It is grown in South America, Indonesia, China, India, and Malaysia.

Since ancient times, patchouli has been highly valued in the Eastern world. It was used to fragrance clothing and linens. When it arrived in the West in the 19th century, paisley shawls were scented with it. In the 1960s, hippies wore it alone as a sign of peace and love, and it is still widely utilized in current perfumery.

The scent of the essential oil is strong and enduring, with notes of wood, earth, and sweetness. When used more liberally, it sedates and stimulates in short doses. Antiseptic and anti-inflammatory, it is.

It is used in aromatherapy to treat eczema, burns, tension, fatigue, and greasy skin and scalp. It's a sensuous, heady oil.

Use: compress, poultice, inhalation, massage, and baths. It works well for an oily-skin facial, a therapeutic head and scalp massage, and a body massage that is either calming or invigorating. When used sparingly in the bath, a few drops will excite; when used more heavily, they will sedate.

Caution: As long as patchouli essential oil is diluted before application, it is completely safe to use at home.

Peppermint (Mentha Piperita)

The herb's fresh or partially dried leaves and blossoms are used to extract oil. Although it grows everywhere, the plant is cultivated in China, Europe, America, and Britain.

Mint has long been valued in China and Japan, and it has even been discovered in 1000 BC Egyptian tombs. In the past, individuals chewed the leaves or drank the tea to treat "nerve or stomach complaints."

Because over one-third of the essential oil is menthol, it stimulates, clears the brain, invigorates, and has a calming, refreshing, and cooling effect.

It works wonders in aromatherapy for headaches, tension headaches, mental exhaustion, muscle aches, varicose veins, sunburns, bug bites, nausea, indigestion, and hot flashes associated with menopause.

Use: compress, inhale, massage, and take a bath. A few drops on a tissue will help reduce headaches and nausea from travel or morning sickness, as well as clear your head whether you're feeling under the weather or just mentally exhausted. Foot fatigue can be relieved with four drops in a basin. Use sparingly in the bath or for massages.

Caution: Because mint essential oil is so strong, avoid applying it directly to your skin right before bed. Use moderation at all times.

Petitgrain (Citrus Auantium Amara)

The bitter orange tree's leaves and twigs are used to extract oil. It is currently grown for commercial use in South America, North Africa, and France.

For centuries, eau de Cologne has used petitgrain due to its revitalizing, energizing, and deodorizing properties. It is now used as a drink flavoring, in cosmetics, and in fragrance.

The essential oil combines invigorating and soothing qualities, and it smells crisp and sour like oranges. It is perfect as a treatment for fatigue or stress of any kind.

Aromatherapy works well for healing a variety of conditions, including anxiousness, back pain, exhaustion, poor energy, and sleeplessness.

Use: Inhalation, massage, and baths. Add the essential oil to a warm bath to help relieve insomnia or unwind after a stressful day. Massage the temples, nape of the neck, upper back, and lower spine to release stress. Moreover, breathe in a few drops from a tissue for immediate relief from stress or exhaustion.

Caution: Using petitgrain essential oil at home is completely safe. Citrus oils should be kept in a dark, cool place to ensure their freshness.

Pine - Longleaf (Pinus Palustris)

The tree's twigs, cones, and needles are all used to extract oil. North America and northern Europe are the commercial growing regions for it.

Pine was utilized for respiratory issues and aches in the muscles by the ancient Greeks and Romans, and it's still used in Scandinavian saunas. To keep illnesses and insects away and to rid rooms of germs, the needles were burned.

The essential oil is invigorating and antimicrobial, with a potent, balsamic, camphorous scent reminiscent of crushed pine needles.

It works wonders as a powerful tonic and germ-killer in aromatherapy, and it's great for viral illnesses like the flu, rheumatism, and coughs as well as for aches and pains in the muscles.

Use: Poultice, inhalation, massage, and baths. Apply pressure to the chest to relieve a cough or blocked nose. Apply to sore spots on your joints. It eases muscle soreness and increases circulation when taken in the bath. When applied directly to a rag, it functions as a potent home disinfectant, ideal for dampening down bathrooms and freshening up shoes.

Caution: Pine essential oil is completely safe to use at home as long as it is well diluted before usage.

Rose (Rosa Damascenea, Rosa Centifolia)

The freshly plucked rose petals are used to extract oil. Although it grows all over the world, it is mostly grown in France, Morocco, Bulgaria, China, and India.

Rose was given as gifts to loved ones, was adored by the gods, was the subject of poetry, and still makes even the most hardened nose tingle. Rosewater was believed by the Romans to drive out hangovers and to prolong orgies with its enticing aroma.

The fragrance of the essential oil is just as lovely as the blossom. They are both so adored that they have an instantaneous, uplifting, and constructive impact.

Aromatherapy treats headaches, sleeplessness, depression, and stress. Rose is great for skin, especially for dryness, wrinkles, puffiness, and broken veins.

Use: Inhalation, massage, and baths. This oil is perfect for scenting a place because it exudes a happy, pleasurable, and romantic atmosphere.

Apply it to your entire body or face during massages, and add ten drops to your bath to help you recover from a difficult day or to help with hangovers.

Caution: If you dilute rose essential oil before using it, it's completely safe to use at home.

Rosemary (Rosmarinus Officinalis)

The evergreen shrub's flowering tops are used to extract oil. China, California, England, and the Mediterranean region all grow it economically.

For a very long time, rosemary was considered a holy herb. Most ancient civilizations included it in their diets and used it for magic and medicine. Burning it helps eliminate infections; eating it helps with liver and digestive issues; inhaling it helps with respiratory and neurological issues.

The essential oil is antibacterial, stimulating, astringent, invigorating, and cleansing. It smells fresh, green, woodsy, and minty.

It is used in aromatherapy to treat dandruff, headaches, respiratory issues, fluid retention, and poor circulation.

Use: Inhalation, massage, and baths. It works especially well as a warm body massage for any aches in the muscles or as a head and scalp massage for headaches, greasiness, and loss of concentration. For physical or mental exhaustion, add it to the bath, and for coughs, bronchitis, and other respiratory issues, inhale it.

Caution: As long as the essential oil of rosemary is well diluted before usage, it is completely safe to use at home. On the other hand, avoid using it if you are pregnant or if you have epilepsy (or if you are massaging someone who does).

Rosewood (Aniba Rosaeodora)

The wood of the tropical evergreen tree is used to extract oil. It's grown for commercial purposes in Peru and Brazil.

Rosewood was highly prized for its aromatic wood, which was especially useful for English furniture from the 19th century. The Amazonian Indians applied it topically to treat skin conditions and wounds. These days, wood is used to make chopsticks, as well as to flavor food and beverages and as an ingredient in some soaps and cosmetics.

The essential oil smells sweet, flowery, and woodsy and has a calming, tonic, healing, relaxing, and slightly sensuous effect. It is also deodorizing.

Aromatherapy works well for every type of skin condition, including dull, dry complexions, wrinkles, scars, and acne. It's a really private and calming oil.

Use: Inhalation, massage, and baths. From a facial to a full body massage, it instantly improves mood and skin. Men and women both enjoy it when used to baths to balance out other oils. It also works wonderfully as a cozy, calming room aroma.

Caution: If diluted before application, rosewood essential oil is completely safe for usage at home.

Sage - Clary (Caliva Sclarea)

The perennial herb's leaves and flowering tips are used to extract oil. Morocco, England, France, and other countries around the Mediterranean grow it for oil.

Once considered one of the most valuable herbs, clary sage was used to treat mental illnesses, infertility, and stomach issues. The herb "clary," which means "clear eye" in Latin, earned its name from its ability to make a calming, restorative eye ointment.

The essential oil smells aromatic, green, and balsamic. It is warming, calming, and gently antiseptic.

Pre-menstrual tension, menstrual cramps, depression, exhaustion, stress, migraines, and skin irritations or inflammations might all benefit from aromatherapy.

Use: Baths and massages. A few drops in the bath will provide you energy and relieve backache, sprains and aches, cramps, low mood, and itchy skin. It works well for massages of the face, neck, and scalp to relieve tension and headaches.

Caution: As long as clary sage is well diluted before application, it is completely safe to use at home. But avoid using it when you are pregnant.

Sandalwood (Santalum Album)

The tree's heartwood and roots are used to extract oil. Although it is also grown in Malaysia, Sri Lanka, and Indonesia, the majority of oil originates from India.

Sandalwood has always been a popular component in perfumes; the ancient Chinese, Indians, and Egyptians used it for embalming and incense. It has been used medicinally to treat skin inflammations and facilitate mucus discharge.

The essential oil is considered an aphrodisiac and has a deep fruity-sweet, woodsy smell. It is also astringent, calming, sedative, and antibacterial.

Aromatherapy uses it to treat emotional issues, tension, sadness, libido loss, sleeplessness, and chapped or damaged skin. It works well as an expectorant for colds and coughs.

Use: compress, inhale, massage, and take a bath. A few drops in a hot bath provide one of the most sensual and calming soaks that can help to detoxify the body and mind. It makes the most calming massage oil and works especially well on dry, rough skin regions. It relieves congestion when applied topically or inhaled while steaming.

Caution: If diluted before application, sandalwood essential oil is completely safe for usage at home.

Spruce (Tsuga Canadensis)

The big evergreen tree's twigs and needles are used to extract oil. It is endemic to North America's west coast, where it is widely grown for oil.

American Indians used the hemlock spruce as medicine. To treat fever and infection, they burnt the branches and prepared a tisane from the bark. The leather industry uses a tannin extract from the bark today.

The essential oil is antibacterial, warming, astringent, soothing, peaceful, and relaxing. It smells clean, fresh, sweet, and balsamic.

Aromatherapy uses it for rheumatism, cellulite, sprains, stiffness and discomfort, poor circulation, coughs, colds, and to ease tension and anxiety.

Use: Poultice, inhalation, massage, and baths. Apply as a heated poultice or dilute and rub into sore, tight, or overworked muscles as a linament. It provides a warming, cellulite-reducing, and circulation-boosting massage for the legs and feet during the winter. It is wonderfully calming and has a sedative effect when taken in the bath. When used with steam, it eases the congestion that accompanies a cold and promotes restful sleep.

Caution: As long as spruce essential oil is well diluted before usage, it is completely safe for use at home.

Tarragon (Artemisia Dracunculus)

The bushy perennial plant's leaves are used to extract oil. Though it is widely farmed, America, Holland, and France produce the majority of the oil.

In the Middle East, tarragon was used to treat flatulence. It was reputed to offer protection from the fangs of crazy dogs, dragons, and other creatures when the Crusaders brought it to Europe! These days, it's utilized to flavor food and condiments.

The essential oil smells strongly like fennel or anise with a hint of green spice. It has sedative, antibacterial, antispasmodic, digestive, and mild diuretic properties.

Aromatherapy can help with a wide range of stomach issues, including constipation, indigestion, gas, premenstrual tension, cramps, and nervous butterflies or knots in the stomach.

Use: compress, massage, and poultice. If you have any stomach issues, massage the abdomen with the well-diluted essential oil using slow, clockwise palm strokes. A hot poultice steeped in the oil can be applied for cramps, wind, or indigestion. It is not advised to use it in the bathtub.

Caution: When used sparingly and with proper dilution, tarragon essential oil is completely safe for domestic usage. But avoid using it when you are pregnant.

Tea-Tree (Melaleuca Alternifolia)

The shrub's leaves and twigs are used to extract oil. All of Australia's oil is produced there; it is native.

The crew of Captain Cook gave the tea-tree its name when they brewed the tiny, black leaves and used them in place of tea. The Aborigines employed it for its amazing healing abilities. Medics were aware of its potent antibacterial and germicidal properties during World War II.

The essential oil is a potent, non-irritating antiseptic that kills germs, fungus, and viruses 12 times more effectively than carbolic. It smells spicy, peppery, and medicinal, like nutmeg.

It is used in aromatherapy to treat diaper rash, cuts, burns, acne, stings, blisters, and herpes. For the treatment of fungal and yeast infections, it works incredibly well.

Use: Poultice, inhalation, massage, and baths. An rapid at-home first aid kit can be created by diluting one part essential oil to nine parts carrier oil. Apply to other irritations such as stings, wounds, burns, and spots. Use it as a douche for fungus or viral illnesses, or add it to the bath.

Caution: If diluted before application, tea-tree essential oil is completely safe for usage at home.

Thyme - White (Thymus Vulgaris)

The perennial herbaceous plant's leaves and flowering tips, either fresh or dried, are used to extract oil. Spain, Morocco, France, Algeria, Israel, and Greece all grow it for oil.

Thyme was used medicinally by the Greeks and Romans, and for embalming by the Egyptians. It is claimed to have been sewed onto knights' armor and placed to the hay in the cot of the infant Jesus to keep them courageous in battle.

The essential oil smells sour and herbaceous and includes thymol, a potent antibacterial. It works well as an insect repellant, expectorant, and stimulant.

Aromatherapy works well for rheumatic aches and pains, tension, exhaustion, anxiety, headaches, skin irritations, and colds and coughs. Most flying insects don't like it.

Use: Inhalation, massage, and baths. When combined with other stress-relieving oils, it creates a revitalizing bath. For headaches, rheumatic pain, and sore muscles, massaging it in is beneficial. When inhaled with steam, it does wonders for respiratory issues.

Caution: If white thyme is carefully diluted before application and used sparingly, it is completely safe to use at home. Don't use it while pregnant, though. Since red thyme is poisonous, it should never be used.

Valerian (Valeriana Fauriei)

The perennial herb's roots are used to extract oil. England, Belgium, France, and Holland grow it for oil.

Throughout Europe, valerian has long been revered as a medicinal panacea. It was stuffed into pillows to help women fall asleep and soothe themselves when they couldn't sleep, and it was put in sickrooms to hasten healing, uplift the mood, and ease discomfort.

The essential oil smells warm, mossy, musky, and woodsy. It is also tranquil, hypnotic, and peaceful.

It works wonders in aromatherapy to relieve stress, anxiety, depression, moodiness, and irritability.

Use: Inhalation, massage, and baths. Either adults or children can be sedated at night by placing a few drops on a tissue next to a pillow. Calming and hypnotic, especially in a warm bath. Additionally, it treats irritability, sleeplessness, and negative moods when used to a calm, relaxing massage.

Caution: As long as the essential oil is sufficiently diluted before application and used sparingly, Valerian essential oil is completely safe to use at home.

Violet (Viola Odorata)

The perennial plant's fresh leaves and blossoms are used to extract oil. China, Italy, and southern France cultivate it for oil.

The fragrant leaves and blossoms have long been used for therapeutic purposes. The plant was utilized as a brightener and skin-soother. They drank tisane to ease headaches and anxieties.

The essential oil is anti-inflammatory, astringent, antibacterial, circulation-boosting, calming, light, and refreshing. It also has a delicate floral and strong green-leaf mix.

Any skin irritation or inflammation can benefit from aromatherapy, but in particular, rashes, thread veins, open pores, acne, blackheads, eczema, spots, and eczema. Additionally, it clears the skull, increases focus, and cures migraines, vertigo, and emotional upheaval.

Use: Inhalation, massage, and baths. Use it for any type of beautifying facial massage. After diluting it, use it to the skin in the morning and evening to revitalize any complexion. After a day of focus, a few drops in the bath will make you a quick thinker with clarity. Additionally, it will ease headaches and emotional distress.

Caution: Violet essential oil is completely safe to use at home as long as it is diluted first.

Yarrow (Achillea Millefolium)

The dried herb's leaves and blooms are used to extract oil. Commercial cultivation of it occurs in America, Africa, France, and Germany.

A traditional remedy for infections, fevers, and stomach issues is yarrow. It is said that the Greek warrior Achilles used it to treat combat wounds before being shot in the heel, which was his one weak point. These days, vermouths are made bitterer by adding it.

The essential oil is anti-inflammatory, antibacterial, astringent, sedative, and profoundly calming. It smells fresh and mossy like camphor.

Aromatherapy can help with blood pressure reduction, nerve relaxation, insomnia treatment, and other stress-related issues. Additionally, it works wonders for rashes, scars, acne, oiliness, and hair health promotion.

Use: Inhalation, massage, and baths. When combined with other calming oils, it works well as a massage oil to ease insomnia. It helps lower blood pressure and soothe anxiety when inhaled via a tissue or diffused into a space. Use a few drops as a toning treatment for your face or to soothe skin when added to a bath.

Caution: As long as yarrow essential oil is well diluted before usage, it is completely safe for use at home. But avoid using it when you are pregnant.

Ylang-Ylang (Cananga Odorata)

The newly gathered blossom of the tropical tree is used to extract oil. Madagascar, the Philippines, and Reunion Island are the commercial growing regions for it.

Tropical Asian islanders used ylang-ylang to cure insect bites, irritated skin, shield their hair, and prevent fever or infection. The Victorians were the first to commercially utilize it in Macassar hair oil, which served as an early conditioner and growth-stimulator. The flower has long been associated with love because of its alluring scent.

The aroma of the essential oil is sweet and strong, like narcissus or hyacinth. Aromatic, hypnotic, and calming, it mostly affects the mind and emotions rather than the physical body. It also revitalizes hair and skin.

It is helpful in aromatherapy to reduce stress, elevate depressed emotions, and heighten sexuality.

Use: Inhalation, massage, and baths. It is best used sparingly because of how strong and pleasant it smells. A few drops in your bath or massage will uplift your spirits, reduce stress, and awaken your senses. Without being sedative, it is among the greatest oils for soothing and relaxing.

Caution: As long as ylang-ylang essential oil is carefully diluted before application and used sparingly, it is completely safe to use at home.

Conclusion

Congratulations, you made it to the end!

I hope you enjoyed the trip we took together in the wonderful and healing world of essential oils as much as I enjoyed sharing my knowledge with you.

The world of essential oils is as vast and versatile as the fragrances they offer. Through the pages of this book, we've embarked on a journey to understand their origins, properties, and the myriad ways they can enhance our lives. From the invigorating scent of peppermint to the calming embrace of lavender, each oil holds the potential to alleviate discomforts, uplift spirits, and foster a deeper connection with nature.

As we've explored the various uses of essential oils for personal care, beauty products, and household cleaning, it's become evident that their benefits extend far beyond mere aromatics. They are potent tools for holistic well-being, offering natural solutions that complement our body's own healing mechanisms.

For those who have found intrigue and inspiration within these pages, I invite you to delve deeper into the world of natural wellness. In my companion book, "Traditional Herbal Remedies and Healing Herbal Teas," (ISBN n. 9781739665241o) you'll discover an array of herbal remedies that further complement and expand upon the principles explored here. Whether you're seeking to soothe aches, enhance relaxation, or simply nourish your body and soul, this guide offers invaluable insights into the healing power of herbs.

May this journey with essential oils and natural remedies serve as a catalyst for greater self-care, mindfulness, and vitality in your life. Let us continue to embrace the wisdom of nature as we nurture ourselves and our surroundings with care and gratitude.

Thank you again for joining me on this aromatic adventure and I hope to meet you again in my next book.

Namastè

Essential Oils Mixing Chart

X = Ok to Mix

Mixing Essential Oils	Ambrette Seed	Angelica	Basil	Bay	Bergamot	Birch White	Camphor White	Cedarwood Atlas	Chamomile German
Ambrette Seed		X			X				
Angelica	X								X
Basil					X				
Bay					X	X	X	X	
Bergamot	X		X	X				X	X
Birch White				X					
Camphor White					X			X	
Cedarwood Atlas				X	X		X		X
Chamomile German		X			X			X	
Citronella	X	X	X		X		X		
Cypress			X	X	X	X	X	X	X
Eucalyptus	X	X	X	X				X	X
Fennel					X	X		X	X
Frankincense			X				X	X	X
Galbanum		X			X				X
Geranium	X	X	X		X	X		X	X
Ginger	X		X	X	X		X		
Jasmine					X			X	X
Juniper	X		X		X	X		X	X
Laurel							X		
Lavender	X	X	X	X	X			X	X

Mixing Essential Oils	Ambrette Seed	Angelica	Basil	Bay	Bergamot	Birch White	Camphor White	Cedarwood Atlas	Chamomile German
Lemon	X		X	X	X	X		X	X
Lemongrass			X			X			
Lime	X		X		X		X	X	
Mandarin	X								X
Marigold Calendula									
Marjoram			X		X				X
Mimosa		X			X				X
Myrrh							X		
Neroli		X			X			X	X
Orange	X				X			X	
Patchouli					X				X
Peppermint	X		X		X		X	X	
Petitgrain	X		X		X				
Pine Longleaf	X		X			X	X	X	X
Rose		X			X				X
Rosemary	X		X	X	X		X	X	X
Rosewood		X			X				
Sage Clary			X		X			X	
Sandalwood				X	X				X
Spruce	X		X						X
Tarragon			X			X	X		
Tea-Tree					X		X		
Thyme White	X		X		X	X			X
Valerian									X
Violet									

Mixing Essential Oils	Ambrette Seed	Angelica	Basil	Bay	Bergamot	Birch White	Camphor White	Cedarwood Atlas	Chamomile German
Yarrow									X
Ylan-Ylang			X		X				

Mixing essential Oils (continued)	Citronella	Cypress	Eucalyptus	Fennel	Frankincense	Galbanum	Geranium	Ginger	Jasmine	Juniper
Ambrette Seed	X		X				X	X		X
Angelica	X		X			X	X			
Basil	X	X	X		X		X	X		X
Bay		X	X					X		
Bergamot	X	X		X		X	X	X	X	X
Birch White		X		X			X			X
Camphor White	X	X			X			X		
Cedarwood Atlas		X	X	X	X		X		X	X
Chamomile German		X	X	X	X	X	X		X	X
Citronella		X					X	X		
Cypress	X		X	X	X		X			X
Eucalyptus		X		X	X		X	X		X
Fennel		X	X		X	X	X	X		X
Frankincense		X	X	X		X	X	X		X
Galbanum	X			X	X		X			
Geranium		X	X	X	X	X			X	X
Ginger	X		X	X	X				X	
Jasmine							X	X		
Juniper		X	X	X	X		X			
Laurel		X	X					X		X

Mixing essential Oils (continued)	Citronella	Cypress	Eucalyptus	Fennel	Frankincense	Galbanum	Geranium	Ginger	Jasmine	Juniper
Lavender	X	X	X	X	X	X	X		X	X
Lemon	X	X	X	X	X		X		X	
Lemongrass	X				X		X		X	
Lime	X	X			X		X			
Mandarin					X	X	X			
Marigold Calendula	X	X								X
Marjoram	X		X				X	X		X
Mimosa					X	X	X		X	
Myrrh		X			X					X
Neroli	X				X	X	X	X		X
Orange					X	X	X	X		
Patchouli	X	X			X		X	X	X	
Peppermint			X	X			X			X
Petitgrain										X
Pine Longleaf		X	X		X					
Rose	X	X		X	X	X	X	X	X	X
Rosemary		X	X	X	X		X	X		X
Rosewood						X	X		X	
Sage Clary		X	X		X		X	X	X	X
Sandalwood		X	X	X	X		X	X	X	X
Spruce			X					X		X
Tarragon										
Tea-Tree			X				X			
Thyme White			X							

Mixing essential Oils (continued)	Citronella	Cypress	Eucalyptus	Fennel	Frankincense	Galbanum	Geranium	Ginger	Jasmine	Juniper
Valerian				X			X			
Violet					X	X	X			X
Yarrow										
Ylan-Ylang					X		X	X	X	X

Mixing essential Oils (continued)	Laurel	Lavender	Lemon	Lemongrass	Lime	Mandarin	Marigold Calendula	Marjoram	Mimosa
Ambrette Seed		X	X		X	X			
Angelica		X							X
Basil		X	X	X	X			X	
Bay		X	X						
Bergamot		X	X		X			X	X
Birch White			X						
Camphor White	X				X				
Cedarwood Atlas		X	X		X				
Chamomile German		X	X			X		X	X
Citronella		X	X	X	X		X		
Cypress	X	X	X		X		X		
Eucalyptus	X	X	X					X	
Fennel		X	X						
Frankincense		X	X	X	X	X			X
Galbanum		X				X			X
Geranium		X	X	X	X	X		X	X
Ginger	X							X	

Mixing essential Oils (continued)	Laurel	Lavender	Lemon	Lemongrass	Lime	Mandarin	Marigold Calendula	Marjoram	Mimosa
Jasmine		X	X	X					X
Juniper	X	X	X				X		
Laurel			X					X	
Lavender			X	X	X	X	X	X	X
Lemon	X	X			X		X	X	
Lemongrass		X						X	
Lime		X	X				X		
Mandarin		X							
Marigold Calendula		X	X		X				
Marjoram	X	X	X	X					
Mimosa		X				X			
Myrrh		X	X						X
Neroli		X	X			X		X	X
Orange		X	X	X	X	X			X
Patchouli		X	X			X			X
Peppermint		X	X						X
Petitgrain		X	X			X			
Pine Longleaf	X	X	X						
Rose		X	X			X		X	X
Rosemary	X	X	X	X	X	X	X	X	X
Rosewood		X	X				X		
Sage Clary		X	X	X	X	X		X	
Sandalwood		X	X				X	X	X
Spruce			X					X	

Mixing essential Oils (continued)	Laurel	Lavender	Lemon	Lemongrass	Lime	Mandarin	Marigold Calendula	Marjoram	Mimosa
Tarragon				X					
Tea-Tree		X	X						
Thyme White		X	X						
Valerian		X							
Violet		X				X	X	X	
Yarrow									
Ylan-Ylang		X	X			X		X	X

Mixing essential Oils (continued)	Myrrh	Neroli	Orange	Patchouli	Peppermint	Petitgrain	Pine Longleaf	Rose	Rosemary
Ambrette Seed			X		X	X	X		X
Angelica		X						X	
Basil					X	X	X		X
Bay									
Bergamot		X	X	X	X	X	X	X	X
Birch White							X		
Camphor White	X				X		X		X
Cedarwood Atlas		X	X		X		X		X
Chamomile German		X		X				X	X
Citronella		X		X				X	
Cypress	X			X			X	X	X
Eucalyptus					X	X	X		X
Fennel					X			X	X
Frankincense	X	X	X	X			X	X	X
Galbanum		X	X					X	

Mixing essential Oils (continued)	Myrrh	Neroli	Orange	Patchouli	Peppermint	Petitgrain	Pine Longleaf	Rose	Rosemary
Geranium		X	X	X	X			X	X
Ginger		X	X	X				X	X
Jasmine				X				X	
Juniper	X	X			X	X		X	X
Laurel							X		X
Lavender	X	X	X	X	X	X	X	X	X
Lemon		X	X	X	X	X	X	X	X
Lemongrass				X					X
Lime						X			X
Mandarin	X	X	X	X		X		X	X
Marigold Calendula									X
Marjoram		X						X	X
Mimosa	X	X	X	X	X			X	X
Myrrh		X	X	X	X			X	
Neroli	X		X	X				X	X
Orange		X		X		X	X		X
Patchouli	X	X	X		X		X		
Peppermint	X			X				X	X
Petitgrain			X						X
Pine Longleaf			X	X					X
Rose	X	X		X	X				
Rosemary		X	X		X	X	X		
Rosewood		X	X					X	X
Sage Clary			X	X	X			X	

Mixing essential Oils (continued)	Myrrh	Neroli	Orange	Patchouli	Peppermint	Petitgrain	Pine Longleaf	Rose	Rosemary
Sandalwood	X	X	X	X	X	X		X	X
Spruce	X						X		X
Tarragon									
Tea-Tree							X		
Thyme White									X
Valerian	X	X	X						
Violet									
Yarrow	X	X	X			X		X	
Ylang-Ylang		X		X		X	X	X	

Mixing essential Oils (continued)	Rosewood	Sage Clary	Sandalwood	Spruce	Tarragon	Tea-Tree	Thyme White	Valerian	Violet	Yarrow	Ylang-Ylang
Ambrette Seed				X			X				
Angelica	X								X		
Basil		X		X	X		X				X
Bay	X		X								
Bergamot	X	X	X			X	X				X
Birch White					X		X				
Camphor White					X	X					
Cedarwood Atlas		X						X			
Chamomile German			X	X			X	X		X	
Citronella									X		
Cypress		X	X								

Mixing essential Oils (continued)	Rosewood	Sage Clary	Sandalwood	Spruce	Tarragon	Tea-Tree	Thyme White	Valerian	Violet	Yarrow	Ylang-Ylang
Eucalyptus		X	X	X		X	X				
Fennel		X						X			
Frankincense		X	X							X	X
Galbanum	X								X	X	
Geranium	X	X	X			X		X	X	X	X
Ginger		X	X	X							X
Jasmine	X	X	X								X
Juniper		X	X	X						X	X
Laurel											
Lavender	X	X	X			X	X	X	X	X	X
Lemon	X		X	X		X	X				X
Lemongrass		X			X				X		
Lime									X		
Mandarin		X							X	X	X
Marigold Calendula	X		X						X	X	
Marjoram		X	X	X						X	X
Mimosa			X						X		X
Myrrh			X	X				X		X	
Neroli	X		X					X		X	X
Orange	X	X	X					X		X	
Patchouli		X	X								X
Peppermint		X	X								
Petitgrain			X							X	X

Mixing essential Oils (continued)	Rosewood	Sage Clary	Sandalwood	Spruce	Tarragon	Tea-Tree	Thyme White	Valerian	Violet	Yarrow	Ylang-Ylang
Pine Longleaf				X		X					
Rose	X	X	X						X	X	X
Rosemary	X		X	X			X				
Rosewood			X								X
Sage Clary			X							X	X
Sandalwood	X	X				X					X
Spruce							X				
Tarragon											
Tea-Tree			X								
Thyme White		X		X							
Valerian											X
Violet											
Yarrow		X							X		
Ylang-Ylang	X	X	X					X	X		

Essential Oils For Common Problems Chart

X = Ok for the Problem

T = Therapeutic

S = Stimulating & Uplifting

R = Relaxing & Calming

Essential Oils For Common Problems	Acne	Anxiety	Arthritis	Atlethe's Foot	Backache	Bites & Stings	Breathing difficulties	Bruises	Bunions	Burns
Ambrette Seed R-S		X	X		X					
Angelica T-R							X			
Basil S						X				
Bay T-S					X					
Bergamot R-S	X	X								
Birch White T				X						
Camphor White S-T					X			X		
Cedarwood Atlas T-S	X						X			
Chamomile German R	X		X			X				X
Citronella T-S					X	X				
Cypress T			X					X	X	

Essential Oils For Common Problems	Acne	Anxiety	Arthritis	Atlethe's Foot	Backache	Bites & Stings	Breathing difficulties	Bruises	Bunions	Burns
Eucalyptus S-T			X		X		X			
Fennel S										
Frankincense R		X								
Galbanum R		X								
Geranium S-R	X			X				X		X
Ginger S-T			X							
Jasmine R		X								
Juniper R-T	X		X		X					
Laurel R-T					X					
Lavender S-R	X	X	X	X	X	X		X		X
Lemon S	X		X						X	
Lemongrass T-S	X			X						
Lime S			X							
Mandarin R		X								
Marigold Calendula T						X		X		X
Marjoram m R-T			X		X		X	X		
Mimosa R		X								
Myrrh S-R			X				X			
Neroli R		X								
Orange S-R										

244

Essential Oils For Common Problems	Acne	Anxiety	Arthritis	Atlethe's Foot	Backache	Bites & Stings	Breathing difficulties	Bruises	Bunions	Burns
Patchouli R-S	X	X								X
Peppermint T-S			X			X	X		X	
Petitgrain S-R	X	X			X					
Pine Longleaf S			X		X		X			
Rose R										X
Rosemary T-S			X		X		X			
Rosewood R	X	X								
Sage Clary R-S		X			X			X		
Sandalwood R	X	X					X			
Spruce R-S		X	X		X					
Tarragon T										
Tea-Tree S-T	X			X		X	X		X	X
Thyme White S-T					X					
Valerian T-R		X								
Violet S		X								
Yarrow R	X									
Ylan-Ylang R		X								

Essential Oils For Common Problems (Continued)	Cellulite	Chicken Pox	Chilblains	Poor Circulation	Cold	Cough	Cramps	Cuts & Abrasions	Dandruff	Depression
Ambrette Seed R-S										
Angelica T-R					X	X				
Basil S				X						
Bay T-S	X				X				X	
Bergamot R-S		X						X		X
Birch White T										
Camphor White S-T					X					
Cedarwood Atlas T-S	X			X		X			X	
Chamomile German R		X					X	X		
Citronella T-S								X		
Cypress T	X		X	X		X				
Eucalyptus S-T		X	X		X	X	X			
Fennel S	X									
Frankincense R						X				X
Galbanum R	X									
Geranium S-R								X	X	X
Ginger S-T			X	X		X				
Jasmine R							X			X
Juniper R-T	X		X	X			X		X	

Essential Oils For Common Problems (Continued)	Cellulite	Chicken Pox	Chilblains	Poor Circulation	Cold	Cough	Cramps	Cuts & Abrasions	Dandruff	Depression
Laurel R-T					X		X			
Lavender S-R	X	X		X	X		X	X	X	X
Lemon S	X		X	X	X	X	X		X	
Lemongrass T-S			X	X	X					
Lime S	X			X	X					
Mandarin R							X			
Marigold Calendula T				X				X		
Marjoram R-T			X				X			
Mimosa R										X
Myrrh S-R				X	X	X				X
Neroli R							X			X
Orange S-R										
Patchouli R-S									X	
Peppermint T-S				X	X	X				
Petitgrain S-R										
Pine Longleaf S				X	X	X				
Rose R							X			X
Rosemary T-S	X		X	X		X			X	
Rosewood R										X

Essential Oils For Common Problems (Continued)	Cellulite	Chicken Pox	Chilblains	Poor Circulation	Cold	Cough	Cramps	Cuts & Abrasions	Dandruff	Depression
Sage Clary R-S				X						X
Sandalwood R	X						X		X	X
Spruce R-S			X	X	X	X				
Tarragon T	X						X			
Tea-Tree S-T		X	X		X			X	X	
Thyme White S-T					X	X				
Valerian T-R										
Violet S										X
Yarrow R										
Ylan-Ylang R				X			X			X

Essential Oils For Common Problems (Continued)	Dermatitis, Psoriasis & Eczema	Fatigue	Fluid Retention	Hair	Hangover	Headache	Herpes	House Cleansers	Indigestion	Influenza
Ambrette Seed R-S		X				X			X	
Angelica T-R									X	
Basil S		X								
Bay T-S				X						
Bergamot R-S	X	X		X			X	X		
Birch White T	X		X							
Camphor White S-T										

Essential Oils For Common Problems (Continued)	Dermatitis, Psoriasis & Eczema	Fatigue	Fluid Retention	Hair	Hangover	Headache	Herpes	House Cleansers	Indigestion	Influenza
Cedarwood Atlas T-S				X						
Chamomile German R	X			X		X	X	X		
Citronella T-S								X		
Cypress T	X		X	X						
Eucalyptus S-T		X				X	X	X		X
Fennel S			X							
Frankincense R						X			X	
Galbanum R		X								
Geranium S-R	X	X	X	X	X			X		
Ginger S-T		X								
Jasmine R		X								
Juniper R-T			X							
Laurel R-T										X
Lavender S-R	X	X		X	X	X	X	X	X	
Lemon S				X	X		X	X		
Lemongrass T-S		X				X		X		
Lime S								X		X
Mandarin R			X						X	

Essential Oils For Common Problems (Continued)	Dermatitis, Psoriasis & Eczema	Fatigue	Fluid Retention	Hair	Hangover	Headache	Herpes	House Cleansers	Indigestion	Influenza
Marigold Calendula T	X						X			
Marjoram R-T									X	X
Mimosa R										
Myrrh S-R	X									
Neroli R					X					
Orange S-R		X								X
Patchouli R-S	X	X	X				X			
Peppermint T-S		X			X	X		X	X	X
Petitgrain S-R		X								
Pine Longleaf S								X		X
Rose R	X				X	X				
Rosemary T-S		X	X	X		X				X
Rosewood R										
Sage Clary R-S		X		X		X				
Sandalwood R	X									
Spruce R-S			X							X
Tarragon T									X	
Tea-Tree S-T				X			X	X		X

Essential Oils For Common Problems (Continued)	Dermatitis, Psoriasis & Eczema	Fatigue	Fluid Retention	Hair	Hangover	Headache	Herpes	House Cleansers	Indigestion	Influenza
Thyme White S-T		X				X		X		X
Valerian T-R										
Violet S	X					X				
Yarrow R				X						
Ylan-Ylang R				X						

Essential Oils For Common Problems (Continued)	Insect Repellant	Insomnia	Jetlag	Measles	Menopause	Nausea	Perspiration	Pre-Menstrual Tension
Ambrette Seed R-S								
Angelica T-R								
Basil S		X						
Bay T-S								
Bergamot R-S				X			X	X
Birch White T								
Camphor White S-T	X							
Cedarwood Atlas T-S								
Chamomile German R		X		X	X			X
Citronella T-S	X						X	
Cypress T		X	X		X			
Eucalyptus S-T				X				
Fennel S								X

Essential Oils For Common Problems (Continued)	Insect Repellant	Insomnia	Jetlag	Measles	Menopause	Nausea	Perspiration	Pre-Menstrual Tension
Frankincense R								
Galbanum R								
Geranium S-R		X	X		X			X
Ginger S-T						X		
Jasmine R		X						X
Juniper R-T								X
Laurel R-T								X
Lavender S-R		X	X	X	X		X	X
Lemon S						X		
Lemongrass T-S	X						X	
Lime S								
Mandarin R		X				X		
Marigold Calendula T								
Marjoram R-T								
Mimosa R		X						
Myrrh S-R								
Neroli R		X						
Orange S-R								
Patchouli R-S								
Peppermint T-S			X		X	X		X
Petitgrain S-R		X						
Pine Longleaf S								
Rose R		X			X			X

Essential Oils For Common Problems (Continued)	Insect Repellant	Insomnia	Jetlag	Measles	Menopause	Nausea	Perspiration	Pre-Menstrual Tension
Rosemary T-S								
Rosewood R								
Sage Clary R-S					X			X
Sandalwood R		X						X
Spruce R-S								
Tarragon T					X			X
Tea-Tree S-T	X			X				
Thyme White S-T	X						X	
Valerian T-R		X						
Violet S								
Yarrow R		X						
Ylan-Ylang R		X			X			

Essential Oils For Common Problems	Rheumatism	Sexual Issues	Skin	Stress	Sunburn	Thrush, Candida & Fungal Issues	Travel Sickness
Ambrette Seed R-S							
Angelica T-R	X						
Basil S				X			
Bay T-S							
Bergamot R-S			X	X			X
Birch White T	X						
Camphor White S-T							
Cedarwood Atlas T-S							

253

Essential Oils For Common Problems	Rheumatism	Sexual Issues	Skin	Stress	Sunburn	Thrush, Candida & Fungal Issues	Travel Sickness
Chamomile German R	X		X	X	X		
Citronella T-S							
Cypress T	X		X				
Eucalyptus S-T	X						
Fennel S							
Frankincense R			X				
Galbanum R			X				
Geranium S-R		X	X	X	X		
Ginger S-T	X	X					X
Jasmine R		X	X	X			
Juniper R-T	X		X			X	
Laurel R-T							
Lavender S-R	X		X	X	X	X	
Lemon S	X		X				X
Lemongrass T-S			X				
Lime S	X		X				
Mandarin R			X				X
Marigold Calendula T			X				
Marjoram R-T	X			X			
Mimosa R			X	X			
Myrrh S-R			X			X	
Neroli R		X	X	X			
Orange S-R			X		X		

Essential Oils For Common Problems	Rheumatism	Sexual Issues	Skin	Stress	Sunburn	Thrush, Candida & Fungal Issues	Travel Sickness
Patchouli R-S		X	X	X			
Peppermint T-S							X
Petitgrain S-R			X	X			
Pine Longleaf S	X						
Rose R		X	X	X	X		
Rosemary T-S	X		X				
Rosewood R		X	X	X			
Sage Clary R-S		X		X			
Sandalwood R		X	X	X		X	
Spruce R-S	X			X			
Tarragon T							
Tea-Tree S-T			X			X	
Thyme White S-T	X		X				
Valerian T-R				X			
Violet S			X				
Yarrow R			X	X			
Ylan-Ylang R		X	X	X			

www.ingramcontent.com/pod-product-compliance
Lightning Source LLC
Chambersburg PA
CBHW01174020426
42333CB00022B/2714